ABC OF
RHEUMATOLOGY

ABC OF
RHEUMATOLOGY

edited by

MICHAEL L SNAITH MD FRCP

Senior lecturer in rheumatology, Institute for Bone and Joint Medicine, University of Sheffield

BMJ
Publishing
Group

First published in 1996
Reprinted 1997
by the BMJ Publishing Group, BMA House, Tavistock Square,
London WCIH 9JR

Third impression 1997

British Library Cataloguing in Publication Data

A catalogue record for this book is available from the
British Library

ISBN 0-7279-0997-5

Typeset by Apek Typesetters Ltd., Nailsea, Bristol
Printed and bound by Craft Print, Singapore

Contents

Preface

This ABC is aimed at a wide range of medical practitioners. I hope that family doctors will find it useful to have available on the premises. For hospital based doctors, it should supplement the more detailed knowledge required by candidates for the MRCP (part 1) with a flavour of everyday practice. There is also some coverage of that rather grey area of medical practice which lies between the provinces of the surgeon and the physician, which is often referred to as orthopaedic medicine and which does not feature in textbooks of internal medicine.

Specialist members of the rheumatology team include nurses, physiotherapists, and occupational therapists. Their contributions are referred to in several chapters, and covered in detail in chapter 19. Surgical appliance fitters are also frequented by patients with arthritis, but not exclusively so. Foot problems are so common, whether or not they presage a systemic rheumatic condition, that I thought they required a chapter, written by podiatrists.

The book initially takes a regional approach, in terms of the common rheumatic problems of the hand, shoulder, and back. These are then followed by a more conventional coverage of syndromes or classified disorders. The series published in the *British Medical Journal* did not include two chapters, which were reserved for the bound volume: Epidemiology and Laboratory Investigations.

Readers of the journal may feel that they need not buy the book, if they have already extracted the chapters: not so! Apart from the additional material already referred to, most of the authors have modified their chapters in response to letters and comments, only some of which were published in the correspondence columns of the *BMJ*.

I should like to express my appreciation to all the authors, to Deborah Reece, commissioning editor and to Greg Cotton, technical editor, for all their forbearance. I would also like to thank the Arthritis and Rheumatism Council for their financial support.

1 PAIN IN THE HAND AND WRIST

Michael Shipley

General considerations

Causes of pain in hand and wrist

At all ages

Trauma
Flexor tenosynovitis
Trigger finger or thumb
Carpal tunnel syndrome
De Quervain's tenosynovitis
Ganglion
Dorsal tenosynovitis
Inflammatory arthritis
Raynaud's syndrome
Reflex sympathetic dystrophy
Chronic upper limb pain
Scaphoid fracture

Elderly patients

Nodal osteoarthritis:
 Distal interphalangeal
 First carpometacarpal
 Proximal interphalangeal
Scaphoid fracture
Pseudogout
Gout:
 Acute
 Chronic tophaceous
Dupuytren's contracture
Diabetic stiff hand

Patients presenting with pain in the hand are often anxious. The hands are so important for daily activities and for communication and contact that any actual or perceived threat to their normal function is worrying. For those whose livings are made by intricate use of their hands—musicians, craft workers, keyboard operators—and for heavy labourers, the threat is often greater. More often than not, people can live with their present pain if their fear of future loss of function can be allayed.

Nature of pain

Localised or diffuse
Unilateral or bilateral
Aching or sharp
Present only with use
Present constantly
Worse at night or at rest
Associated with sensory symptoms

Assessment

Patients' descriptions of their pain are important. Its quality, localisation, variability with rest or use, and the presence of any associated symptoms such as numbness or pins and needles will often be diagnostic. Trauma, sometimes unnoticed, is the most common cause of hand pain. Specific diagnoses vary slightly with age.

Pain in the hand and wrist may reflect a problem arising proximally; the rest of the arm and the neck should always be examined, as should the other hand. Severe pain in the hand may seem to spread up the arm to the axilla or neck. Neck pain on the same side may be primary or reflect muscle spasm, resulting from holding the arm immobile in order to protect it. Several systemic disorders—most commonly inflammatory arthritis—may present as hand pain, usually bilateral, and a full locomotor and general examination is necessary.

Injection technique

Hand and arm well supported
Equipment readily to hand
Clean skin thoroughly
Use small bore needle
Inject small volume of local anaesthetic
Inject corticosteroid through same needle
Always inject under low pressure

Treatment

Physiotherapy helps some patients, but locally applied gels of non-steroidal anti-inflammatory drugs are of only limited value. Oral non-steroidal anti-inflammatory drugs should be used with care when the problem is localised because the risk of side effects may outweigh the severity of the problem and the potential benefit.

Problems may resolve spontaneously, but the main treatment for many patients is a local injection—local anaesthetics not containing adrenaline followed by 0·2–1 ml of a suitable corticosteroid preparation, such as hydrocortisone acetate 25 mg/ml and triamcinolone hexacetonide 20 mg/ml (which is about five times as powerful as hydrocortisone on a mg/ml basis). Patients should be warned that the pain often increases for a day or so after injection. There may be some leakage of the corticosteroid back along the needle track when the injection site is superficial. This may cause local depigmentation of skin and atrophy of subcutaneous fat. This risk is considerably increased when depot corticosteroid preparations are used.

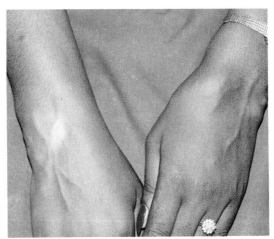

Skin depigmentation caused by superficial injection of depot corticosteroid.

1

Tendon problems

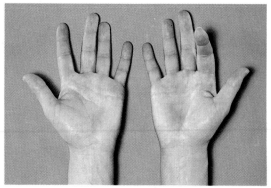

Flexor tenosynovitis.

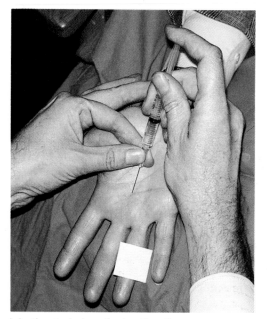

Injection technique for treating flexor
tenosynovitis or trigger finger.

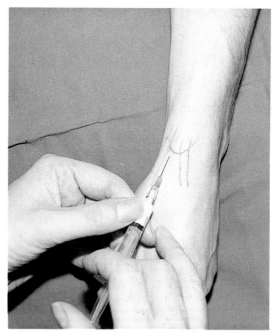

Injection technique for treating De Quervain's
tenosynovitis.

Flexor tenosynovitis

Inflammation of tendon sheaths in the hand causes stiffness and pain
of one or more fingers, usually worse in the morning. Thickening of the
affected tendon sheaths in the palm is diagnostic. Swelling may be
mainly just proximal to the wrist or over the proximal phalanges and
into the palm. Typically the affected finger cannot be fully extended,
and active flexion is more limited than passive flexion.

Treatment—If, after a brief period of rest, treatment is still indicated
patients should be given a local injection from the palmar approach
along the line of the tendon. Under local anaesthesia, corticosteroid
(10–20 mg hydrocortisone, or 5–10 mg triamcinolone in more severe
cases or if hydrocortisone fails) is injected into the tendon sheath or
adjacent to it, under low pressure to ensure that it is not being injected
into the tendon itself.

Trigger finger or thumb

The development of tendon nodules is common with rheumatoid
arthritis and is a complication of diabetes mellitus, but it can occur
spontaneously. The nodule can be palpated and moves with the flexor
tendon. It causes local pain or triggering—the finger becomes fixed in
flexion because of the nodule jamming on the proximal side of a pulley
and has to be flicked straight. Rarely, irreversible flexion may develop.

Treatment—A local injection of corticosteroid is the treatment of
choice; it should be injected into the region of the nodule, and
preferably into the tendon sheath, under low pressure (not into the
nodule itself). The technique is the same as for flexor tenosynovitis.

De Quervain's tenosynovitis

This problem is related to use. It causes pain around or just proximal
or distal to the radial styloid at the point where the abductor pollicis
longus tendon runs over the radial styloid and under the extensor
retinaculum. There is local tenderness and swelling; the pain can be
reproduced by forced flexion of the thumb into the palm or by active
abduction of the thumb against resistance. In elderly patients it is
distinguished from osteoarthritis of the first carpometacarpal joint by
the more proximal site of the pain.

Treatment—A resting splint that immobilises the thumb may help,
but the quickest treatment is to inject 25 mg hydrocortisone or 10 mg
triamcinolone. Under local anaesthesia, the needle is inserted along the
line of the tendon, just proximal or distal to the styloid, at the site of
maximum tenderness. Injection under low pressure beside the tendon
will produce palpable swelling of the tendon sheath.

Dorsal tenosynovitis

Inflammation of the extensor tendon sheath generally reflects an
underlying inflammatory arthritis. The swelling bulges to either side of
the extensor retinaculum of the wrist to produce an hourglass swelling.
Treatment is by injection of corticosteroid.

Ganglion

This is a bulge or tear of the synovial lining of a joint or tendon
sheath and is filled with gelatinous fluid. It occurs around the wrist and
is non-inflammatory and generally painless. The swelling is firm or
occasionally fluctuant. Ganglia usually resolve spontaneously but
occasionally require aspiration with a wide bore needle. Recurrence is
common, and surgical excision may be necessary.

Dupuytren's contracture

This is a painless thickening of the palmar aponeurosis that produces
gradual flexion, initially of the little and ring fingers. The overlying
skin is puckered and, unlike flexor tenosynovitis, does not move when
the finger is flexed. If the fixed flexion is disabling, excision by a
specialist is advisable.

Carpal tunnel syndrome

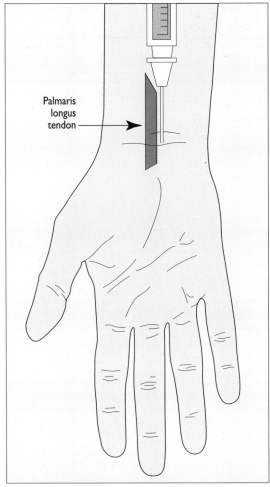

Palmaris
longus
tendon

Injection technique for treating carpal tunnel syndrome.

This is the commonest cause of hand pain at night. It is caused by flexor tenosynovitis, premenstrual retention of fluid, or the later stages of pregnancy. It is also common with rheumatoid arthritis and may be the presenting feature. It causes any combination of pain, numbness, pins and needles, and a sense of swelling. The symptoms are brought on by daytime use of the hand in some patients. It is characterised by the median nerve distribution of the symptoms—the pins and needles are sharply localised to the radial three and a half digits—but if the pain is severe it may be difficult for patients to localise the symptoms. Such patients may need an outline drawing of the hand to mark out their night time distribution of pins and needles. A wrist splint worn at night will often relieve pain and pins and needles and, if so, is diagnostic. Nerve conduction studies are useful to confirm the diagnosis if it is uncertain and to determine the severity of the nerve damage. A negative test does not absolutely rule out the syndrome but calls it into question.

Treatment

In milder cases a splint worn at night for a few weeks is curative. Weight loss may help, but diuretics do not. If the symptoms are not relieved but do not justify surgery a local injection of corticosteroid is usually helpful. If symptoms persist surgical decompression should be performed without delay to prevent persistent numbness and wasting of the thenar muscles.

Injecting the carpal tunnel—The hand is placed comfortably palm up, and a fine needle is inserted into the proximal palmar crease just to the ulnar side of the palmaris longus tendon or about 5 mm to the ulnar side of the tendon of the flexor carpi radialis. The needle is inserted at an angle of 45° to the skin and aimed towards the palm. Under local anaesthesia the needle is advanced gently. If the needle is in the nerve initial injection will cause immediate pain in the fingers, showing that the needle must be repositioned. Once the needle is correctly sited corticosteroid is injected slowly (initially 25 mg hydrocortisone or, if this fails, 10–20 mg triamcinolone). The symptoms may be induced briefly towards the end of the injection, and the patient should wear a resting splint for the next few days.

Nodal osteoarthritis

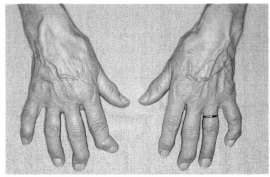

Nodal osteoarthritis with Heberden's nodes.

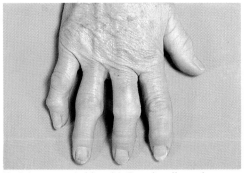

Nodal osteoarthritis with Bouchard's nodes.

Nodal osteoarthritis may develop painlessly or with an initial acute phase that produces local pain, swelling, and redness. The latter may cause confusion and lead to misdiagnosis as rheumatoid arthritis. Nodal osteoarthritis is uncommon before the age of 45, and there is often a family history of the condition. Once the acute phase has settled (usually in a few weeks or months) the pain and redness subside, but bony swellings remain. These swellings are called Heberden's nodes when the distal interphalangeal joints are affected and Bouchard's nodes when the proximal interphalangeal joints are affected. Nodal osteoarthritis may coexist with other hand problems. Reassurance that the pain will settle and that function is little affected in the long term is usually sufficient treatment. Although the effects of nodal osteoarthritis are unsightly, surgery is not recommended.

First carpometacarpal osteoarthritis may present with acute pain and swelling at the base of the thumb. The joint is tender, and there may be crepitus. During this acute phase an injection of 10 mg hydrocortisone into the joint may help, as may immobilisation in a splint. Usually the pain settles spontaneously, leaving a prominent stiff joint and an adducted thumb—the square hand of osteoarthritis. Surgical intervention is helpful if pain persists.

Systemic disorders causing hand pain

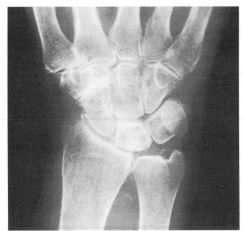

Chondrocalcinosis in wrist.

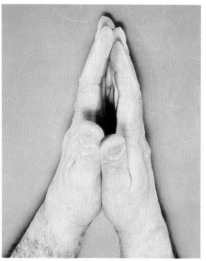

Cyanosis seen in Raynaud's phenomenon.

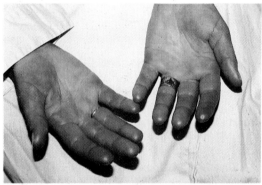

Positive prayer sign of diabetic stiff hand.

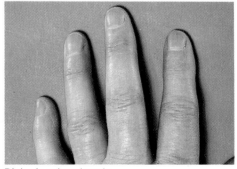

Diabetic sclerodactyly.

Inflammatory arthritis

The hand is a common site for the first signs of rheumatoid arthritis or of an inflammatory arthritis associated with psoriasis (it is less commonly affected by ankylosing spondylitis or reactive arthritis). The pattern of involvement is usually characteristic; symmetrical involvement of the proximal interphalangeal and metacarpophalangeal joints suggests rheumatoid arthritis, while dactylitis (synovitis of the joint and tendon sheath, with or without cutaneous psoriasis) is often associated with psoriasis or other causes of a seronegative arthritis. An acute onset of nodal osteoarthritis can mimic these symptoms, but osteoarthritis can coexist with an inflammatory arthritis.

Crystal synovitis of the wrist

Acute pseudogout—An acutely inflamed wrist in an elderly patient is occasionally due to synovitis induced by calcium pyrophosphate crystals. Chondrocalcinosis can be seen in radiographs, usually on the ulnar side of the wrist. Chondrocalcinosis increases in prevalence with age and is generally asymptomatic, but it can be the diagnostic feature of this acutely painful inflammatory arthritis. Although technically difficult, aspiration of joint fluid from the wrist reveals turbid fluid containing calcium pyrophosphate crystals, which are weakly positively birefringent. A short course of non-steroidal anti-inflammatory drugs will control the symptoms. Frequent attacks require regular rather than intermittent treatment with such drugs.

Acute gout—Sodium urate crystals can induce synovitis of the wrist or finger joints, particularly in elderly patients who are taking diuretics or who have been admitted to hospital. In such cases the gout may be polyarticular. The symptoms may closely mimic those of acute rheumatoid arthritis. Fluid from the affected joint contains crystals of sodium urate that are strongly negatively birefringent, and the serum urate concentration is usually raised. An acute attack should be treated with non-steroidal anti-inflammatory drugs or, if these are contraindicated, with colchicine (1 mg immediately and then 0·5 mg every six to eight hours). Chronic tophaceous gout is relatively painless but may produce severe deformity of the hand. Allopurinol should never be used to treat an acute attack but may be needed if attacks are frequent or when tophi are present.

Raynaud's phenomenon

This is an undue vasospastic response of the digital artery to cold. The fingers develop pallor followed by cyanosis and then by painful redness due to rebound hyperaemia—the triphasic response. This is a primary and harmless problem in young women in their teens or early 20s. A secondary form, usually coming on later in life, may be a manifestation of rheumatoid arthritis, systemic lupus erythematosus, or scleroderma. It also occurs as an industrial disease in people who use vibrating tools. Avoidance of cold is usually sufficient treatment, but occasionally vasodilator drugs are necessary.

Diabetic stiff hand

Diabetic patients may develop a stiff, painful hand and the so called positive prayer sign. Diabetic sclerodactyly produces tight, shiny skin. Its cause is unknown, but it is commoner in poorly controlled diabetes and may be a marker of vascular complications of diabetes. Other problems that may contribute to stiffness of hands include flexor tenosynovitis, Dupuytren's contracture, and nodal osteoarthritis.

Other disorders

Scaphoid bone fracture

This is caused by a fall onto an outstretched arm with the wrist in dorsiflexion. There is pain, swelling, and tenderness in the anatomical snuff box at the base of the thumb. The symptoms may be mild and can be overlooked unless the possibility of a fracture is considered. Diagnosis is made by x ray: a series of four scaphoid views will show most fractures, but if there is doubt a repeat series two weeks later or a bone scan may be necessary.

Treatment—There is debate about the best treatment for scaphoid fractures, but most units treat undisplaced fractures by immobilisation for six to eight weeks with a below elbow cast enclosing the thumb. For displaced fractures and those that show signs of delayed union, internal fixation and possibly bone grafting should be considered.

Reflex sympathetic dystrophy (Sudeck's atrophy)

This condition may follow trauma, surgery, or a stroke. The cause is unknown. In the arm the hand and wrist are most commonly affected. Patients develop burning pain, hyperaesthesia, stiffness, and puffiness in the affected part. The skin becomes reddened, smooth, and glossy, and there is increased sweating. Radiographs show patchy osteoporosis of the hand.

Treatment—Most patients recover spontaneously but will do so more quickly if they are given adequate pain relief and are encouraged to move the affected hand despite the pain. Severe cases should be referred to a specialist pain centre. About half of patients are helped by a guanethidine block of the affected limb.

Chronic (work related) upper limb pain syndrome

This is the preferred name for repetitive strain injury, "teno," and associated disorders in which the predominant symptom is pain in all or part of one or both arms with no easily discernible cause. The problem is often work related and has achieved a degree of notoriety because of the severity of the symptoms with few physical signs. People are often severely distressed, and there may be obvious disharmony at their place of work. The syndrome is particularly prevalent among people who work for long periods without breaks at repetitive keyboard jobs. Musicians may have similar problems and can be greatly helped by expert advice on their playing technique. The pathology is unclear, but increased muscle tension, heightened awareness of normal or increased sensory nerve input, and anxiety driven introspection are all possible contributing factors.

Treatment—It is helpful to be objective and non-judgmental, discussing the cause of the problem as a combination of physical and psychosocial factors without assuming which is primary. A substantial reduction in use of the arm for a defined period, a gradual return to work, and the help of a sympathetic but firm physiotherapist will usually resolve the problem. Patients' employers should be encouraged to review the content of their job and the layout of the work place and to be positive and sympathetic. This will help their employees and reduce the risk of litigation.

> An overlooked scaphoid fracture is a common cause of litigation

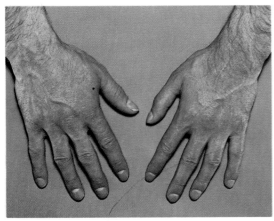

Sudeck's atrophy of right hand.

Characteristics of chronic upper limb pain syndrome

Often starts in hand or wrist
May spread to forearm or arm
Few physical signs but exclude epicondylitis, ganglion, tenosynovitis, etc
Often associated with:
  Repetitive use of keyboard
  Sudden change in work practices
  Disharmony at work
  Anxiety and sleeplessness
Best regarded as having both physical and psychosocial causes
Best dealt with non-judgmentally

The photograph of skin depigmentation was supplied by M L Snaith. The other photographs have been reproduced from Shipley M, ed, *Wolfe coloured atlas of rheumatology* 3rd edition (London: Mosby-Year Book Publishing) 1993 with permission of the publishers.

2 PAIN IN THE NECK, SHOULDER, AND ARM

M Barry, J R Jenner

Neck pain

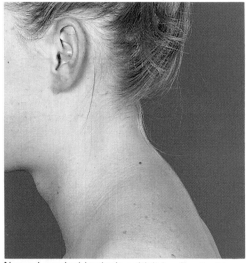

Normal cervical lordosis, which is often lost in neck disorders.

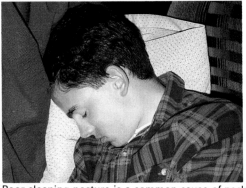

Poor sleeping posture is a common cause of neck pain.

Pain in the neck is a common clinical presentation in primary care and rheumatological practice. It has been estimated that half of the population will have an episode of neck pain during their lifetime. Up to a third of patients attending general practices with neck pain will have had symptoms lasting more than six months or recurring in bouts.

Symptoms arising in the neck are often poorly localised, and there may be difficulty making a precise anatomical diagnosis, particularly as the clinical signs of neck disorders are neither sensitive nor specific. However, certain features of a patient's history and examination help to distinguish common mechanical disorders from more sinister systemic disease. A full history and physical examination are therefore essential for anything other than trivial neck pain.

"Mechanical" disorders

Acute spasm of the neck muscles (spasmodic torticollis) is a common phenomenon. The exact cause of the spasm is uncertain but often appears to be due to bad posture. Examples include poor positioning of a computer screen, inappropriate seating, and sleeping without adequate neck support. Another common offender is carrying unbalanced loads, such as a heavy briefcase or shopping bag. A careful history is often required to identify such factors.

Degenerative changes in the cervical spine (cervical spondylosis) may be associated with neck pain but usually only when the degenerative changes are severe. Mild or moderate degenerative changes are often seen in asymptomatic individuals. In general the pain of mechanical disorders is intermittent and related to use. At least partial relief may be gained by supporting the head and neck.

Neurological changes associated with entrapment of cervical nerve root

Nerve root	Muscle weakness	Reflex changes	Sensory changes
C5	Shoulder abduction and flexion Elbow flexion	Biceps	Lateral arm
C6	Elbow flexion Wrist extension	Biceps Supinator	Lateral forearm Thumb Index finger
C7	Elbow extension Wrist flexion Finger extension	Triceps	Middle finger
C8	Finger flexion	None	Medial side lower forearm Ring and little fingers
T1	Finger abduction and adduction	None	Medial side upper forearm Lower arm

Pain referred to the arm may indicate irritation or entrapment of a nerve root. Common causes are a prolapsed cervical disc or degenerative changes, including apophyseal joint or ligamentous hypertrophy and osteophytes. Neurological examination will often reveal the level of entrapment.

Systemic causes of neck pain

Inflammatory
Ankylosing spondylitis
Rheumatoid arthritis
Polymyalgia rheumatica

Malignancy
Myeloma
Metastatic disease

Infection
Staphylococcal or other sepsis
Tuberculosis

Metabolic
Osteomalacia

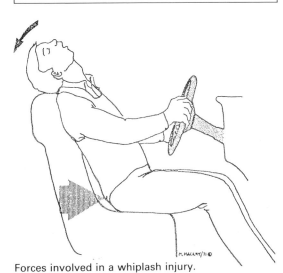
Forces involved in a whiplash injury.

Systemic disease

Inflammatory, neoplastic, or infective disease is suggested by unremitting pain, often radiating to both arms, that is worse at rest and causes considerable sleep disturbance. Neck movements are usually painfully limited in all directions.

Whiplash injuries

Neck injuries sustained in road traffic accidents may occur after front, side, or rear collisions. The start of pain may be delayed for a few hours or even several days after the accident. Restriction of cervical movements may be considerable, but investigation often reveals no pathology. The pain can radiate to the shoulders, arms, and head and is probably caused by stretching or tearing of cervical muscles and ligaments. The principles of treatments are the same as for any acute neck pain, with early mobilisation and avoidance of prolonged use of a collar.

Recovery is often slow, with neck pain persisting beyond six months in up to 10% of patients. Psychological disturbance is often seen in such people, who seem to have coped poorly with their injuries and only slowly revert to their previous level of functioning. The syndrome is related to a number of factors including the stress of having been involved in an accident, frustration at the lack of improvement despite reassurance and treatment, and resentment at prolonged suffering through no fault of their own. In such circumstances a sympathetic approach is important while encouraging patients to take responsibility for their symptoms.

Fibromyalgia

Neck pain and tenderness may be part of a more generalised state of hyperalgesia with multiple tender trigger areas together with general malaise and non-restorative sleep pattern. In the absence of any abnormalities on investigation this condition is referred to as fibromyalgia.

Investigations

Plain *x* rays of the cervical spine are rarely helpful in diagnosing the cause of neck pain except after acute trauma when major injury is suspected. The finding of degenerative changes is common in people aged over 40 and is usually symptomless.

The advent of magnetic resonance imaging has enhanced our ability to diagnose and assess more serious disorders, which include atlantoaxial subluxation in rheumatoid disease, tumours, abscesses, and injuries (such as ruptured ligaments). It can be used to identify prolapsed cervical discs and demonstrates loss of intervertebral disc hydration, but so far it has not revealed the mechanical abnormalities to which we attribute most neck pain.

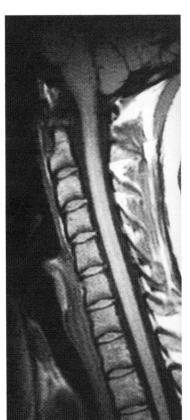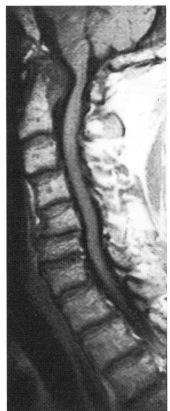
Magnetic resonance images of cervical spine: (left) loss of normal lordosis but no other abnormality; (right) advanced rheumatoid disease of cervical spine, with considerable distortion of lower medulla by pannus around the odontoid peg and gross reversal of normal lordosis at C5, compressing the nerve cord.

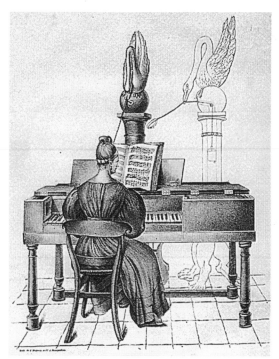

Self traction as recommended by French surgeon Delpech in 1825.

Shoulder pain

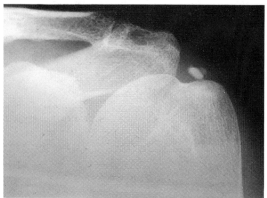

Calcification in rotator cuff.

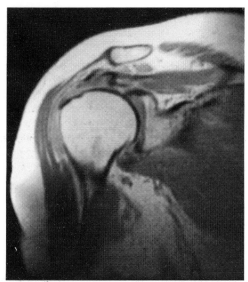

Coronal oblique magnetic resonance image of right shoulder of 50 year old woman with chronic shoulder pain. There is a full thickness tear of supraspinatus tendon with retraction and muscle atrophy.

Treatment

The principles of treatment of acute and chronic neck pain have changed in recent years. Previously, when pain or muscle spasm was intense a period of rest was often prescribed, usually with the patient in a collar. This approach often encouraged the persistence of neck stiffness and disability. Instead, early active treatment is now recommended for neck pain. Collars, if prescribed, should be worn only during activities likely to exacerbate the pain and not used for more than two or three weeks.

Early mobilisation or manipulative techniques aimed at restoring full range of movement are usually helpful. Mobilisation means moving the joint or joints within their restricted range, while manipulation involves moving the joint briefly beyond its restricted range in an attempt to improve range of movement. These treatments are performed by some physiotherapists, by osteopaths and chiropractors, and by some appropriately trained doctors. When manipulation fails traction is sometimes used but is less popular than previously. Autotraction—in which a patient stretches his or her own neck—has long been used and is popular in Scandinavia and the United States but is little used in Britain.

Advice on the correction of postural abnormalities is important in preventing recurrence of pain. Programmes based on the Alexander technique can be helpful when tension and posture seem to be a problem (as with musicians, for example). Radicular pain is treated with rest and wearing a collar for no longer than two weeks. Intractable root symptoms need to be investigated further, and, on the rare occasions that the spinal cord is compromised, a surgical opinion should be sought.

Periarticular disorders

The shoulder is the most mobile joint in the body, but to achieve this mobility it is dependent for stability on surrounding soft tissue structures, in particular the musculo-tendinous rotator cuff. It is therefore not surprising that disorders of the rotator cuff account for most shoulder pain. In patients aged under 40 impingement or tendinitis of the rotator cuff is the commonest problem and usually follows excessive use or trauma. In keeping with most shoulder disorders, pain is felt in the upper arm and the patient is often unable to lie on the affected side at night. The presence of a painful arc on abduction of the arm and pain on resisted movement with localised tenderness of the insertion of the rotator cuff confirms the diagnosis. x Ray pictures of the shoulder occasionally show calcium deposition within the supraspinatus tendon or subacromial bursa, but this is often an incidental finding.

In older patients varying combinations of repeated impingement of the cuff under the acromion, intrinsic degeneration of the cuff, and pressure from bony spurs at the acromioclavicular joint may lead to tears of the rotator cuff. These are either partial or complete and can be associated with chronic and sometimes severe pain.

Pain localised to the top of the shoulder or suprascapular region suggests a disorder of the acromioclavicular joint or neck. Pathology of the acromioclavicular joint is common and is usually traumatic (for example, from playing a sport) or osteoarthritic. Clinical examination reveals tenderness of the joint and pain on passive horizontal adduction. Pain referred to the shoulder tip from diaphragmatic irritation—caused by conditions such as gall bladder disease, subphrenic abscess, and pulmonary embolism—should also be considered.

Causes of a stiff, painful shoulder joint

Adhesive capsulitis
Usually primary
Secondary to diabetes mellitus or intrathoracic pathology

Joint inflammation
Inflammatory arthropathy (such as rheumatoid or psoriatic)
Infection

Osteoarthritis
Secondary to trauma, neuropathic joint, or diabetes

Prolonged immobilisation
Hemiplegia
Strapping after dislocation

Polymyalgia rheumatica

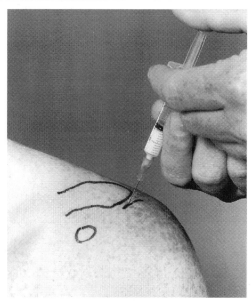

The acromioclavicular joint is often overlooked as a site of shoulder pain and is easily injected.

Glenohumeral disorders

Glenohumeral disorders are classically associated with loss of external rotation. Adhesive capsulitis is characterised by limitation of both active and passive movements of the shoulder with pain at the extremes of motion. Most cases are primary, although the condition may follow a rotator cuff lesion or occur in association with lung disease, myocardial infarction, or stroke. The pathogenesis is unknown. Symptoms may last a year or more, and it is important to reassure patients about the eventual good outcome.

In young people hypermobility of the glenohumeral joint is a commonly unrecognised cause of shoulder pain. It causes aching and a "dead" sensation in the arm that is precipitated by throwing. The shoulder is least stable inferiorly, and a gap may be felt between the acromion and the head of the humerus when the muscles are relaxed— a positive sulcus sign. Intervention other than advice on strengthening exercises is usually not necessary unless instability is severe and leads to recurrent dislocation.

Patients with polymyalgia rheumatica often present with bilateral shoulder pain and stiffness. This may be mistaken for an intrinsic glenohumeral disorder, as polymyalgic symptoms can improve because of systemic absorption of locally injected corticosteroids. Osteoarthritis involving the glenohumeral joint is uncommon as a primary disorder, and if it is present an underlying cause should be sought.

Treatment

Rotator cuff disorders usually respond to rest, non-steroidal anti-inflammatory drugs, and, if persistent, injections of mixtures of corticosteroid preparations and local anaesthetic into the subacromial bursa. Long acting depot preparations of corticosteroids such as methylprednisolone should be used with caution because of the possibility of atrophy of soft tissue or rupture of the tendon if this is injected inadvertently. Tears of the rotator cuff are often managed conservatively, but continuing pain and functional impairment may require either arthroscopic or open repair of the rotator cuff. The acromioclavicular joint is easily palpated and readily accessible for injection.

Treatment of adhesive capsulitis is directed towards giving adequate pain relief, restoring range of movement, and correcting any underlying cause if present. Intra-articular injection of corticosteroid or a short course of oral corticosteroids for two weeks given early in the course of the condition can sometimes help to control pain but does not restore range of movement. The patient should be instructed in stretching exercises when the pain subsides.

Elbow pain (tennis elbow and golfer's elbow)

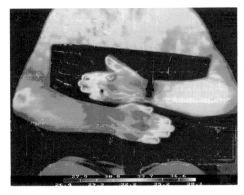

Thermogram of patient with lateral epicondylitis showing "hot spot" over right lateral epicondyle.

Lateral epicondylitis is characterised by variable arm pain aggravated by gripping or twisting movements. Tenderness is greatest over the lateral epicondyle. Useful confirmatory tests are pain on resisted extension of the wrist or on forced radial deviation with the elbow extended. With medial epicondylitis, pain often radiates across the flexor aspect of the forearm. Tenderness over the medial epicondyle and pain on resisted pronation of the wrist confirms the diagnosis. Referred pain from the cervical spine is often felt around the elbow and may mimic soft tissue lesions.

Treatment

Most cases of epicondylitis settle with one or two injections of hydrocortisone acetate mixed with local anaesthetic. Long acting corticosteroids should be used with caution because of the risk of skin atrophy. The injection is often extremely painful for one or two days, and patients should be warned about this. Elbow splints and ultrasound treatment may also be of use. For recurrent epicondylitis, deep massage or frictions can be helpful. Several surgical procedures are described for treating resistant lateral epicondylitis, but none is outstandingly effective.

3 LOW BACK PAIN

J R Jenner, M Barry

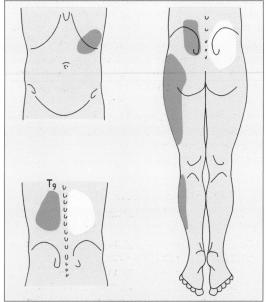

Radiation of pain after injection of 0·1–0·3 ml 6% hypertonic saline into sacrospinal muscle (yellow) and multifidus muscle (red). Note similarity to distribution of sciatic pain.

Low back pain is a major and increasing cause of disability in the United Kingdom. In 1993, 11% of the population reported that their activities had been restricted by back pain within the past four weeks. Satisfactory treatment of low back pain depends on an accurate diagnosis, but finding the cause for low back pain is often not possible because of difficulties in localising the source of the pain.

In 1938 it was shown that many structures in the lumbar spine, when irritated, give rise to pain with very similar distributions. Despite technological advances the identification of an exact source of pain or an exact pathological diagnosis often remains elusive. It is important for doctors and patients to understand that the diagnosis of low back pain therefore depends on identifying some clinical syndromes on the basis of a patient's history and examination, with appropriate investigations to exclude serious pathology and support the clinical diagnosis. If this principle is misunderstood the result can be a misleading diagnosis and inappropriate treatment.

Back pain syndromes

Clinical features of back pain due to mechanical cause

History of pain	Examination
Sudden onset	Asymmetrical lumbar movements
Previous recurrent episodes	Asymmetrical straight leg raise *or*
Unilateral symptoms	Femoral stretch test
Eased by rest	Uniradicular neurological signs

Functional distribution of lumbar nerve roots

Nerve root	Muscle weakness	Reflex changes	Sensation
L2	Hip flexion Hip adduction	None	Front of thigh
L3	Knee extension	Knee	Inner knee
L4	Knee extension Foot dorsiflexion	Knee	Inner shin
L5	Foot inversion Great toe dorsiflexion Knee flexion	None	Outer shin Dorsum of foot
S1	Foot plantar flexion Knee flexion	Ankle	Lateral border of foot and sole

Mechanical back pain or prolapsed lumbar disc

It is vital to distinguish mechanical causes of back pain from other causes as patients with mechanical causes are likely to respond to physical forms of treatment. The symptoms and signs of mechanical back pain differ considerably from those associated with back pain caused by underlying systemic disease.

Most acute episodes of low back pain arise in the triad of joints that allow one vertebra to articulate with another (that is, the intervertebral disc anteriorly and the two facet joints posteriorly). The commonest primary pathology is degeneration of the nucleus pulposus in the lumbar disc. The disc itself is often not the source of pain; this may arise in other structures, such as the facet joints or the many surrounding ligaments, that come under stress as a result of the disc pathology. It is important that doctors explain this to patients so that they understand why just removing their disc will not always cure the pain.

True sciatica, with pain and numbness in the distribution of a single lumbar nerve root, may be accompanied by sensory, motor, or reflex changes and is most commonly caused by a posterolateral protrusion of a disc impinging on the nerve root.

Clinical features of back pain due to systemic cause

History of pain	Examination
Gradual onset and progressive	Stiff or rigid spine
Symmetrical or alternating distribution	Symmetrical restriction of lumbar movements
Worse with rest	Symmetrical restriction of straight leg raising
Disturbs sleep	
Morning stiffness for over 30 minutes	Multiradicular neurological signs

Clinical features of back pain due to spinal stenosis

History of pain	Examination
Leg pain on walking	Stiff spine
Neurogenic claudication	Normal straight leg raising
Eased by leaning forward or sitting but not standing still	Normal peripheral pulses
At ages over 60	Nerve root signs appear late

Common predisposing factors for postural back pain

Postural fault	Cause
Flat lordosis	Seating—car seats, low sofas and armchairs
	Beds—old, soft beds
	Household tasks—ironing, vacuuming, low work surfaces
	Bending—gardening, poor lifting technique
Exaggerated lordosis	Footwear—high heeled shoes
Scoliosis	Unequal leg length—congenital, old leg fracture, running on cambered roads

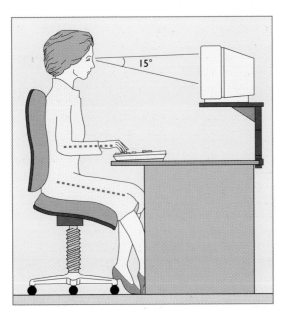

Ideal posture for working at a computer terminal.

Systemic back pain

As well as back pain, there may be associated systemic features such as weight loss, pyrexia, and general malaise. Examination should include the testicles and prostate in male patients and the breasts in female patients as tumours in the sex organs metastasise preferentially to the skeleton.

Ankylosing spondylitis

This can be difficult to distinguish from mechanical pain, especially in the early stages. However, morning stiffness for more than 30 minutes, pain that alternates from side to side of the lumbar spine (a symptom rarely reported in any other cause of back pain), sternocostal pain, and chest expansion of less than 5 cm (less than 2·5 cm for American Rheumatism Association criteria) suggest ankylosing spondylitis. Education, anti-inflammatory drugs, and exercise are the mainstays of treatment.

Spinal stenosis and lateral recess stenosis

Spinal stenosis is common in people aged over 60 and is often not considered in the diagnosis of back and leg pain. It is caused by a narrowing of the spinal canal or intervertebral foramen resulting from degenerative disease. The symptoms should be compared with those of peripheral vascular disease (in this condition the pain eases when a patient stands still and upright). Computed tomography is the investigation of choice. In severe cases surgery may be required to decompress the stenotic area.

Postural pain

Bad posture is probably the commonest cause of persistent back pain. The spine depends for its strength on maintaining a series of arches. Sitting and leaning forward tend to flatten the arch or lordosis, while wearing high heels tends to exaggerate the arch (hyperlordosis or sway back).

Unequal leg length is easily overlooked; 2% of the normal adult population have differences in leg length of at least 2 cm, and such people are more prone to back pain. This can be diagnosed in the surgery by placing wooden blocks of different thicknesses under the short leg and checking the pelvic level visually. Up to a third of patients with back pain and differences in leg length of more than 2 cm will gain relief with a heel raise.

Advice on correcting bad postural habits may be difficult for a patient to accept and may need to be reinforced through programmes such as a back school.

Referred pain

Pathology in organs in the posterior part of the abdominal cavity may refer pain to the back—for example, aortic aneurysm or enlarged lymph nodes. Examination of the abdomen is vital for exclusion of these diagnoses.

Psychological aspects

Symptoms and signs of chronic low back pain in patients with physical disease and abnormal illness behaviour

	Physical disease	Abnormal illness behaviour
Tenderness	Localised	Superficial, widespread, non-anatomical
Axial loading	No lumbar pain	Lumbar pain
Simulated rotation	No lumbar pain	Lumbar pain
Straight leg raising	Limited despite distraction	Improves with distraction
Loss of sensation	Dermatomal	Regional
Loss of power	Myotomal	Regional, jerky, giving way
General response	Appropriate pain	Overt pain response

Some patients' symptoms seem to be exaggerated and disproportionate to the physical signs. A history of involvement in medicolegal proceedings may be obtained. While the possibility of missed pathology must always be borne in mind, examination may reveal inappropriate physical signs.

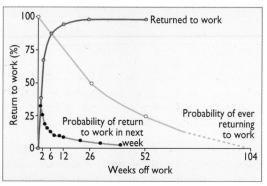

Return to work as a function of time away from work because of back pain.

If a patient has been off work for many months the prognosis is poor; the longer people are off work with low back pain the less likely they are to work again. The reasons for this are unclear but have as much to do with psychological processes as organic pathology. The concept of learned illness behaviour is popular and may explain the persistence of symptoms of chronic unremitting back pain in patients in whom an organic cause cannot be found. This syndrome probably has links with other syndromes such as fibromyalgia and chronic fatigue syndrome.

Investigations

Radiographic evidence of disc infection or vertebral collapse occurs late in the course of a disease, and blood tests are probably a better initial screen for systemic disease.

Blood tests

A blood count, erythrocyte sedimentation rate, and biochemical screen (calcium, phosphate, and alkaline phosphate) should be performed when a systemic cause for back pain is suspected. Testing for prostate specific antigen is useful if prostatic malignancy is suspected.

Radiological investigation

Plain radiographs of the lumbar spine are rarely helpful, particularly when taken early in the course of an episode of back pain, and should be performed only if systemic disease is suspected.

Bone scans are helpful in cases of suspected malignancy and may be abnormal in metabolic bone disease and ankylosing spondylitis.

Other imaging techniques

These should be performed only when initial conservative treatment has failed and surgery is being considered.

Computed tomography is the method of choice for showing bony abnormalities such as bone destruction due to malignancy, infection, or spinal canal stenosis. It can also help in revealing lesions of discs and other soft tissue.

Magnetic resonance imaging is still not widely available but is the investigation of choice for showing lesions of soft tissues, including lumbar disc lesions and tumours.

Radiculography was until recently the standard method for investigating lumbar disc lesions. It is now used only when the level of the lesion is uncertain and magnetic resonance imaging is not available.

Discography is a specialist investigation and may help to identify patients who would benefit from surgical fusion of the spine.

Computed tomogram showing malignant infiltration of lower thoracic vertebra.

Electromyography

A segmental electromyograph may help to confirm the presence of nerve root degeneration if radiological evidence of abnormal anatomy is not conclusive.

Treatment

Bed rest should be kept to a minimum, and early mobilisation should be encouraged

Elements of a back school

Session 1—Principles of anatomy of the spine
Session 2—Applied body mechanics and posture
Session 3—Ergonomics
Session 4—Relaxation techniques and exercises

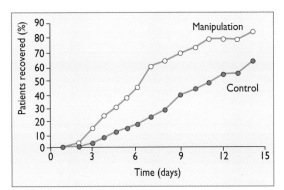

Effect of manipulation on recovery from acute back pain.

Interventional techniques for treating sciatica

Chemonucleolysis—intradiscal injection of proteolytic enzyme
Percutaneous discectomy—by automated nucleotome or laser
Microdiscectomy
Conventional discectomy

The sources of the data presented in illustrations are as follows: J H Kellgren, *Clin Sci* 1939; **4**: 35–46 for the diagram of radiation of pain; G Waddell *et al*, *Spine* 1983; **9**: 209–13 for the box of symptoms and signs of physical illness and abnormal illness behaviour; G Waddell *Spine* 1987; **12**: 632–44 for the graph of return to work after time off because of back pain; and J A Mathews *et al*, *Br J Rheumatol* 1987; **26**: 416–23 for the graph of effect of manipulation on acute back pain. The data are reproduced with permission of the journals.

Treatment should be given early, with the aim of stopping the problem from becoming chronic.

Bed rest

Bed rest has been the main treatment for all forms of acute back pain for many years, with recommendations varying from a few days to over six weeks. The few satisfactory trials that have been published suggest that bed rest for two or three days has the same or greater benefit than longer periods of rest and that shorter bed rest leads to an earlier return to work. Slightly longer periods of rest may be justified for sciatica.

Treatment of low back pain

Patient education and exercise—Reassuring patients, giving them appropriate information, and advising them on posture and exercise programmes are important. These measures are most effective when given as part of a structured programme such as a back school.

Back schools are effective for treating acute back pain. The concept of back schools was developed in Sweden and is based on a series of four sessions, each lasting an hour. Treatment is in groups so that several patients may be treated in one session by a single therapist with no need for specialist facilities. Patients can also benefit from talking with fellow sufferers.

Manipulation has been the subject of many studies, with conflicting results. Manipulation seems to be effective in the first three weeks after the start of acute back pain and gives quicker relief of pain, but after three weeks it may have little advantage over natural recovery. The most effective method is unknown, but physiotherapists, chiropractors, and osteopaths, who use a variety of techniques, all seem effective. Manipulation should not be used with patients with evidence of nerve root entrapment as it may make the root lesion worse.

Treatment of sciatica

Traction—Continuous or intermittent traction remains a popular treatment for patients suffering from sciatica, though recent studies have not consistently confirmed its benefit.

Epidural injections of local anaesthetic and depot preparations of corticosteroid may speed recovery from sciatica. Both the caudal and lumbar routes are used. Depot corticosteroid preparations are not licensed for use in the epidural space, but serious adverse reactions are rare.

Interventional treatments—For patients with symptoms of sciatica lasting more than six weeks despite conservative treatment and in whom the presence of a disc protrusion is confirmed, surgical or chemical removal of the nucleus of the disc should be considered. The success rates for these techniques are 70–80% at one year after treatment, but the rates tend to fall with time, particularly for some surgical techniques.

Chronic low back pain

Once back pain has been established for more than a year the prognosis is poor. Lesions that might be amenable to surgery, such as disc protrusion or spondylolysis, must be excluded. Patients may be referred to a pain clinic for local injections of corticosteroid or cryotherapy to facet joints or sclerosant injections into ligaments, but the success of these procedures for chronic pain is low.

The main aim of treatment should be to help patients to come to terms with their pain and to accept that they can do much themselves to relieve their symptoms. This can be achieved with help from intensive rehabilitation programmes or "schools for bravery," which are available in specialist centres. Treatment, carried out either on a day case basis or as an intensive three to four week inpatient programme, combines physical and psychological approaches to managing back pain.

4 PAIN IN THE HIP AND KNEE

E Paice

Pain in the hip

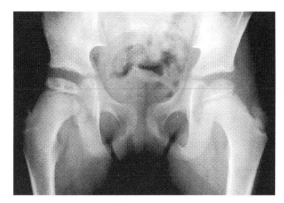

Perthes' disease of right hip.

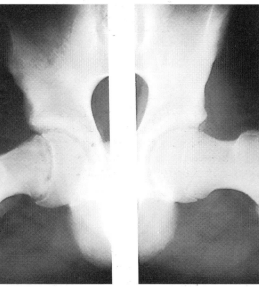

Slipped right femoral epiphysis (epiphysis has slipped down and back in relation to neck of femur).

Hip disease in adults is usually associated with pain on walking or on rolling over in bed, limited movement of the joint, a limping or waddling gait, and shortening of the affected leg. It may be difficult to put on socks and to get up from a low chair.

Irritable hip in childhood

This is a non-specific term for pain in the groin, a limp, and limited movement of the hip joint in all directions in a child. The child should be kept in bed and investigated immediately by general physical examination, plain *x* ray and ultrasound pictures of the hips, full blood count, and measurement of erythrocyte sedimentation rate, with further investigations as necessary to establish a specific diagnosis.

Perthes' disease—Osteochondritis of the epiphysis of the femoral head occurs in boys aged 4–10 years. Plain *x* ray pictures reveal widening of the joint space, narrowing of the epiphysis, and, later, fragmentation of the femoral head. Further deformity of the femoral head may be limited by use of abduction braces or casts.

Infection of the hip joint in a child usually follows bony infection and is rapidly destructive. The child refuses to bear weight on the leg and appears ill. In neonates there are few signs, and the diagnosis is easily missed. *x* Ray changes are late, so if there is clinical suspicion ultrasonography should be carried out to detect an effusion, and any fluid should be aspirated and cultured. An infected hip should be surgically drained and treated with high dose intravenous antibiotics and bed rest.

Slipped epiphysis most often occurs in overweight adolescents. A combination of shearing forces and inherent epiphysial weakness leads to the superior epiphysial plate slipping downward and backward, either suddenly or gradually. There is pain after exertion, and the hip may be held in external rotation. *x* Ray pictures show widening and irregularity of the epiphysis with displacement. Treatment consists of surgical stabilisation of the epiphysis.

Transient synovitis affects children aged under 10 years. It is of unknown aetiology, there are no *x* ray changes (though ultrasonography may reveal an effusion), and the condition resolves within two months.

Juvenile chronic arthritis—The hips are often affected in this condition but usually only after it has affected other joints. It is important to monitor hip movement as contractures may develop insidiously; active physiotherapy and home exercises are needed to prevent deformity.

Infection

Pain is usually the presenting feature with this condition, although systemic features of weight loss, night sweats, and rigors may be prominent. Patients who have pre-existing rheumatoid arthritis or hip prostheses or who are immunocompromised are particularly prone to infection and have fewer systemic manifestations. *x* Ray pictures are often unhelpful at first, and ultrasonography, magnetic resonance imaging, and bone scanning with radioisotopes are more useful. The joint should be aspirated, and the fluid cultured. Treatment consists of surgical drainage, bed rest, and antibiotics.

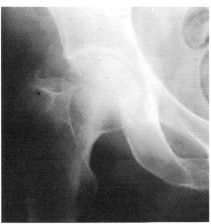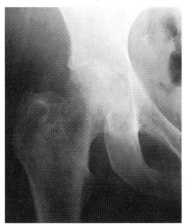

Infected right hip; (left) at presentation and (right) three weeks later.

Causes of pain in hip region

Pain in buttock
- Polymyalgia rheumatica   • Sacroiliitis
- Vascular insufficiency   • Referred from back

Pain in groin
- Diseases of hip joint   • Fracture
- Hernia   • Psoas abscess

Pain in lateral thigh
- Trochanteric bursitis
- Meralgia paraesthetica
- Fascia lata syndrome

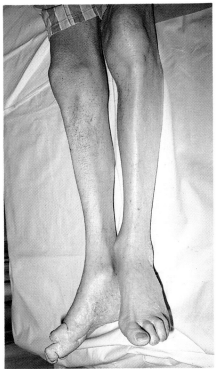

Short, externally rotated left leg from unsuspected hip fracture in patient with rheumatoid arthritis.

When a patient with rheumatoid arthritis suddenly cannot walk suspect fracture of the hip or knee

In chronic inflammatory arthritis the knee is usually affected early while the hip is affected late

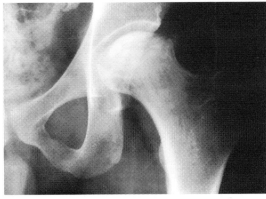

Avascular necrosis of left hip.

Soft tissue problems around hip

Overuse from sports or other activities may cause a variety of soft tissue problems around the hip. The adductor or abductor muscles may be strained, the fascia lata may be inflamed, or there may be inflammation in one of the bursae about the hip (the most commonly affected being the greater trochanteric), causing pain and tenderness in the lateral thigh. A tight iliotibial band crossing the greater trochanter may cause a snapping hip, which may be painful. Footballers' "groin strain" is caused by excessive exertion leading to rupture of muscle or tendon fibres. These conditions are best treated by rest, referral to a physiotherapist, or local corticosteroid injection.

Hip fracture

Fracture of the neck of the femur related to osteoporosis has reached epidemic proportions in elderly women. The diagnosis may not be immediately obvious if there is no history of significant trauma. Unsuspected hip fracture is an important reason for sudden loss of mobility in a patient with rheumatoid arthritis.

Osteoarthritis

Primary osteoarthritis usually presents in people aged over 60. The presenting complaint is of pain, often diffuse and sometimes felt more in the thigh and knee than in the hip itself. At first the pain is relieved by rest, but later it becomes constant. There may be tenderness in the groin over the femoral head. An antalgic gait and fixed flexion deformity of the hip are late signs. Conservative measures such as weight loss, non-steroidal anti-inflammatory drugs, physiotherapy, and a walking stick are useful in the early stages, but later total hip replacement is usually required.

Polymyalgia rheumatica

Patients with this condition usually present with pain in the shoulder girdle, but occasionally the pain and stiffness start in one or both hips, especially the buttocks and thighs. The condition is characterised by severe morning stiffness and gelling after sitting, and the erythrocyte sedimentation rate is usually raised. Corticosteroid treatment is dramatically effective.

Rheumatoid arthritis

The hips are affected in about half of patients with rheumatoid arthritis but usually late in the disease. It is unusual for patients with this condition to present with hip pain. The same is true for the other chronic inflammatory arthritides except for ankylosing spondylitis.

Avascular necrosis

In patients with risk factors for this condition any hip pain should be investigated. x Ray pictures and radioisotope bone scans may both show abnormalities, but magnetic resonance imaging seems to be most sensitive for early changes. Risk factors include treatment with heparin or corticosteroids, systemic lupus erythematosus, a history of exposure to increased barometric pressure, high alcohol consumption, pregnancy, and sickle cell disease.

Malignancy

The hip and pelvis are common sites for secondary bony deposits. The pain of malignancy is likely to be severe and unremitting, present day and night, and accompanied by weight loss. Radioisotope bone scanning is more sensitive than plain x ray for detecting secondary deposits.

Pain in the hip and knee

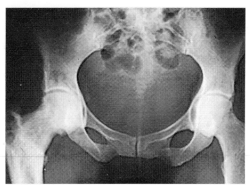
Paget's disease of right hip.

Paget's disease

This disease of elderly people is often associated with osteoarthritis of the hip, and it can be difficult to decide which condition is causing the pain. It is wise to treat the Paget's disease before considering hip replacement. After treatment with calcitonin or bisphosphonates, hip surgery may not be required, and if it is it will certainly be easier to perform.

Osteomalacia

This is most often seen in vegetarian Asian women and in elderly people. There may be an associated proximal myopathy, giving a waddling gait. Looser's zones are seen on x ray pictures. Treatment consists of vitamin D supplements (ergocalciferol).

Pain in the knee

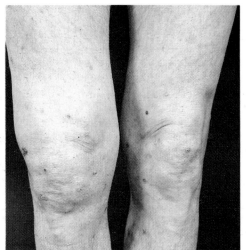
Acutely inflamed knee (urate gout).

Common causes of hot, red, swollen knee

- Infection
- Reiter's disease
- Gout
- Pseudogout

A young man with a hot, red, swollen knee and no history of trauma is most likely to have Reiter's disease

---

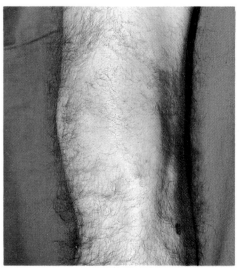
Chronic knee synovitis in patient with psoriasis.

Pain and stiffness in the knee result in a limp and limitation of knee movement. Swelling is best seen in the suprapatellar pouch, and an effusion can be demonstrated by fluctuation or the patellar tap. Stability of the ligaments should always be tested. Pain in the knee may be referred from the hip, pelvis, or lumbar spine, and examination of these should always be included. In adolescents a slipped femoral epiphysis may present as knee pain.

Hot, red, swollen knee

The knee is the most commonly infected joint, and infection must be considered and excluded in every case but especially in patients who are immunocompromised. The infective organism is *Staphylococcus aureus* in 70% of patients, but streptococcal and gonococcal infections also occur. Other conditions to consider are Reiter's disease, gout, and acute calcium pyrophosphate crystal arthritis in elderly people. Trauma may cause an acute synovitis or a haemarthrosis. Occasionally rheumatoid, psoriatic, or juvenile chronic arthritis will present in this way. Fluid should be aspirated by an experienced doctor using an aseptic technique. The fluid should be examined by polarising light microscopy for crystals, Gram staining, and culture for organisms. Blood culture, full blood count, and x rays are indicated.

Chronic inflammation

The knee is commonly affected in most chronic inflammatory arthritides, including rheumatoid arthritis, psoriatic arthritis, and ankylosing spondylitis.

Osteoarthritis

Knee pain in middle aged and elderly people is one of the commonest rheumatic complaints, and an even larger number of people have radiological evidence of knee degeneration. Progression of degeneration is unpredictable, but when pain is persistent and unrelieved by conservative measures, such as anti-inflammatory drugs and exercises, consideration should be given to total knee replacement.

Internal derangements of knee

Mechanical disturbance of the knee usually follows a traumatic incident. The patient may present immediately with a knee effusion, which when aspirated may reveal frank blood. Alternatively, the patient may not present until there have been several episodes of the knee giving way, locking, or swelling. In either case orthopaedic referral is indicated.

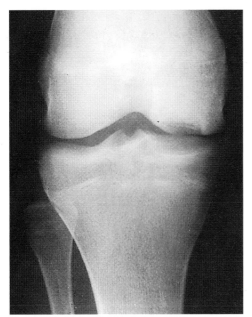

Osteochondritis dissecans of medial femoral condyle.

Osteochondritis dissecans

In this condition a small piece of bone that has become demarcated from the condyle detaches to become a loose body in the joint. Patients are usually aged 15–20 and complain of knee pain and of the knee giving way, locking, or swelling. Surgical intervention may be required.

Anterior knee pain

This is a syndrome of anterior knee pain caused by athletic overactivity, particularly in teenage girls. Walking up or down stairs or sitting with bent knees aggravates the symptoms. The patella is tender on its undersurface. Arthroscopy is indicated in only the most troublesome cases. It may reveal degenerating cartilage on the posterior surface of the patella, in which case the condition is termed chondromalacia patellae. Physiotherapy, strapping, and, occasionally, surgical intervention may be needed.

Osgood-Schlatter disease

This is a problem of athletic adolescents. There is pain and tenderness over the tibial tubercle, which may be swollen. This is a clinical diagnosis, and x ray pictures are not required. The condition usually responds to avoidance of running or kicking for six months.

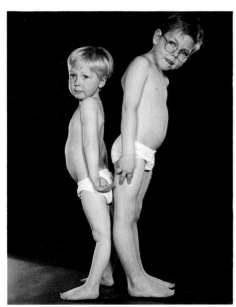

Brothers with knee pains and familial hypermobility. (Reproduced with parents' consent).

Hypermobility

Knee pain related to joint hypermobility is a common problem and may start in childhood. Even without a history of patellar subluxation, recurrent transient knee pain is common and is usually aggravated by such exercise. It is best treated by avoiding activities such as gymnastics and ballet that further stretch the ligaments and by performing isometric exercises.

Growing pains

This term is the name given to a well defined syndrome in children and should only be used in this context. The child wakes in the night with pain in the legs and occasionally the arms. When the limbs are rubbed the pain disappears within minutes. By morning there is no trace of discomfort or disability, and no abnormality is found on examination or investigation. The condition eventually clears up without sequelae.

Medial knee pain

Middle aged and elderly patients may have local tenderness over the medial joint line. This is sometimes called anserine bursitis and is usually relieved by local corticosteroid injection into the tender area.

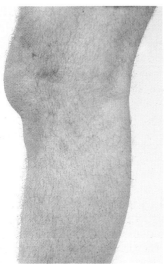

Infected prepatellar bursa in electrician.

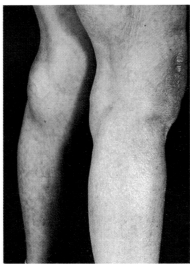

Bilateral popliteal cysts.

Bursae and cysts

Prepatellar bursitis occurs in people whose work involves kneeling and leaning forward, while inflammation of the infrapatellar bursa develops from kneeling upright. If infection is suspected fluid should be removed for culture, otherwise treatment consists of rest. The use of a thick foam cushion to kneel on will help prevent recurrence. A popliteal cyst may cause posterior knee discomfort, which may become acute calf pain if the cyst ruptures. Removal of the cyst is rarely indicated; it is more useful to treat the underlying knee synovitis.

Photographs were prepared by the Photographic Department, Whittington Hospital NHS Trust.

5 PAIN IN THE FOOT

S G West, J Woodburn

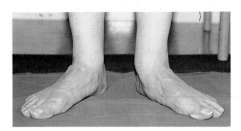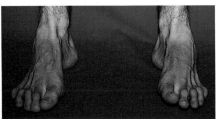

Abnormally pronated feet with Haglund's deformity of heel (left); abnormally supinated feet (right).

Characteristics of the adult foot

Three main types:
- Normal   Pronated (flat)   • Supinated (high arch)

Examination:
- *Examine* the foot when bearing weight and when unloaded
- *Inspect* patient's shoes for abnormal or uneven wear
- *Consult* a podiatrist if a structural or mechanical abnormality is suspected—many can be treated with orthoses

---

Foot pain is common, whether local to the foot or due to systemic disease, mechanical dysfunction, degeneration, or inflammation. In general a multidisciplinary approach to treatment is best, and this is reflected in increasingly close liaison between podiatry, rheumatology, and orthopaedics. Podiatrists (chiropodists) offer a range of treatments from surgery to orthoses. To understand dysfunction, clinicians should be familiar with the normal development and anatomical variants of the foot.

Characteristics of child's foot

Normal foot
- Flexible foot structure (may look flat with a valgus heel)
- Medial longitudinal arch forms when child stands on tiptoe
- Heel to toe walking
- Forefoot in line with rear foot
- Mobile joints with pain free motion and no swelling
- Adopts adult morphology by about 8 years of age

Abnormal foot
- Inflexible   • Rigid valgus (pronated) foot with everted heel position
- High arch foot with toe retraction and tight extensor tendons
- Toe walking   • Delay or difficulty in walking or running
- Abducted or adducted forefoot relative to heel
- Pain, swelling, or stiffness of joints
- Lesser toe deformities   • Hallux deformity

Pain in the forefoot (metatarsalgia)

This is one of the most common forms of foot pain and has several possible causes.

Morton's metatarsalgia (interdigital neuroma)

This normally affects the proximal part of the plantar digital nerve and accompanying plantar digital artery. Trauma to these structures leads to histological changes including inflammatory oedema, microscopic changes in the neurolemma, fibrosis, and, later, degeneration of the nerve. Morton's neuroma is a result of an entrapment lesion of the interdigital nerve.

Clinical features include a gradual onset with sudden attacks of neuralgic pain or paraesthesia during walking, often in the third and fourth toe. Examination may reveal lesser toe deformities and slight splaying of the forefoot, abnormal pronation, and hallux valgus. These often occur in women who wear court shoes. Compression of the cleft or laterally across the metatarsal heads may produce acute pain and the characteristic "Mulder's click."

Treatment—Patients should be advised about suitable footwear and possibly be given orthoses to control abnormal pronation. Injections of local anaesthetic and hydrocortisone around the nerve or surgical excision can be helpful.

Causes of pain in the forefoot

Primary
- Functional and structural forefoot pathologies

Secondary
- Rheumatoid disease • Stress lesions
- Post-traumatic syndromes
- Diabetes • Gout • Paralytic deformity
- Sesamoid pathology • Osteoarthritis

Unrelated to weight distribution
- Nerve root pathology
- Tarsal tunnel nerve compression syndrome—analogous to carpal tunnel syndrome; often misdiagnosed as foot strain or plantar fasciitis; primary symptom is burning feeling on sole of foot in the dermatome served by the medial plantar nerve

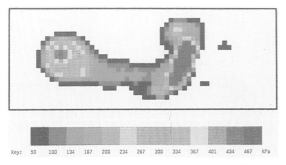

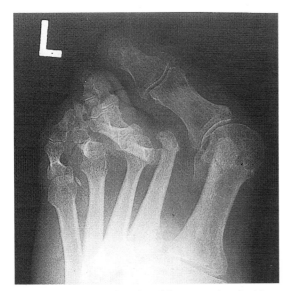

Composite peak pressure profile of right foot of 57 year old woman with rheumatoid arthritis. Note high pressure readings over second, third, and fourth metatarsal heads.

Typical structural deformity of foot associated with diabetic neuropathy.

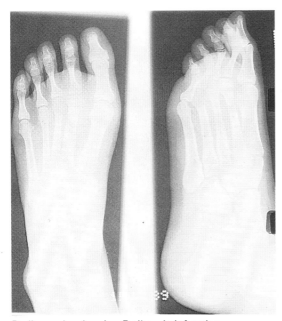

Radiographs showing Freiberg's infraction.

Stress fracture (march fracture)

Associated with increased activity, a stress lesion can affect any of the metatarsal shafts, often along the line of the surgical neck. It can occasionally be seen in patients with osteoporosis as a pathological fracture.

Clinical features—Patients have a history of increased activity, change in occupation or footwear, or sudden weight gain. The symptoms are a dull ache along the affected metatarsal shaft changing to a sharp ache just behind the metatarsal head. The pain is exacerbated by exercise and is more acute at "toe off." There is tenderness and swelling over the dorsal surface of the shaft. Pain is produced by compression of the metatarsal head or traction of the toe. x Rays may not reveal the fracture for two to four weeks, but if it is important to confirm the diagnosis (for example, with an athlete who needs advice on whether to continue sport) a bone scan can reveal it sooner.

Treatment—Rest and local protective padding with partial immobilisation are usually sufficient. These fractures rarely require casting.

Acute synovial effusion

This condition is normally associated with acute trauma, leading to inflammation of the synovial membrane with accompanying effusion. Systemic causes of acute synovitis, such as seen in rheumatoid arthritis, and infection should be excluded when making the diagnosis.

Clinical features—It is rare in children but often affects young adults. Patients complain of a sudden start of painful throbbing that is made worse by movement. There may have been trauma or a systemic inflammatory disorder. Any movement of the joint produces pain. There is a fusiform swelling around the distended joint, and crepitus may be felt.

Treatment—Rest, immobilisation, and ultrasound treatment may help if the cause is trauma. Anti-inflammatory drugs are sometimes helpful. Any hint of previously unsuspected systemic arthritis should be followed up.

Acute inflammation of anterior metatarsal soft tissue pad

This common condition is generally found in middle aged women. It affects the soft tissues of the plantar aspect of the forefoot and is associated with increased shear forces, such as with wearing "slip on" and high heeled court shoes.

Clinical features—Patients present with a burning or throbbing pain localised to the soft tissues anterior to the metatarsal heads. The pain usually develops over a few weeks, is often associated with walking in a particular pair of shoes, and is usually relieved by rest. The tissues are inflamed, warm, and congested. Direct palpation, rotation, and simulation of shear forces on the foot exacerbate the pain. Examination of patients' shoes may reveal a worn insole with a depression under the metatarsal heads.

Management—Advice on footwear, with adequate support or cushioning, should be given. Associated abnormal pronation or lesser toe deformities should be corrected with orthoses.

Osteochondritis (Freiberg's infraction)

This quite common condition generally affects the second or third metatarsal heads. It is an aseptic necrosis or epiphyseal infraction associated with trauma and localised minute thrombosis of the epiphysis.

Clinical features—It affects teenagers and is associated with increased sporting activity. The presenting complaint is often a limp with a dull pain associated with movement of the metatarsal phalangeal joint, exacerbated at toe off. The long term result is a flattened metatarsal head, which can progress to arthritis. The affected joint may be slightly swollen, with a disparity in toe length and width. Traction causes pain. Restricted movement may be due to muscle spasm in the early stages and later to arthritis. Radiographs show distortion of the metatarsal head.

Treatment—In the early stages rest and immobilisation are sufficient, but sometimes patients eventually require corrective surgery.

Pain in the foot

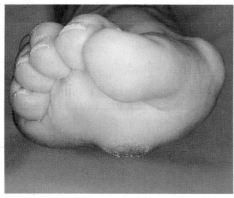

Severe plantar metatarsal bursitis affecting second metatarsal head of patient with rheumatoid arthritis. Overlying callus suggests that this is a high pressure site during normal gait.

Plantar metatarsal bursitis

This condition may affect the deep anatomical or superficial adventitious bursae. In the acute form—such as in dancers, squash players, or skiers—the first metatarsal is usually affected, while the second to fourth metatarsals are affected in chronic inflammatory arthritis.

Clinical features—Patients present with a throbbing pain under a metatarsal head that usually persists at rest and is exacerbated when the area is first loaded. The acute condition affects men and women equally, usually in younger adults. If a superficial bursa is affected there will be signs of acute inflammation, with fluctuant swelling and warmth. With deep bursitis, the tissues are tight and congested. Direct pressure or compression produces pain, as does dorsiflexion of the associated digit.

Treatment—Anti-inflammatory drugs are useful; in practice both local gels and systemic oral drugs help. Injections of corticosteroid may be indicated in severe cases. Patients must rest the affected part, and this may be achieved by protective padding. Any underlying deformity or foot type with abnormal function should be assessed and treated.

Plantar fascia affections

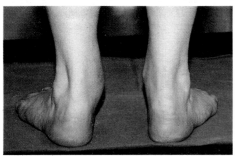

Valgus heel.

Pain along the medial longitudinal arch is quite common. Most affected patients have abnormal foot mechanics, such as abnormal pronation, valgus heel, or a flat foot. Other conditions include true plantar fasciitis, which is characterised by a few fast growing nodules in the fascia, and plantar fibromatosis, which is characterised by fibrous nodules and contracture of the fascia.

Treatment of the true plantar fascial strain requires rest and control of abnormal function with orthoses. Ultrasound treatment may seem helpful, but controlled trials are lacking.

Painful heel

> ### Common causes of painful heel
>
> *Pain within heel*
> Disease of calcaneus—osteomyelitis, tumours, Paget's disease
> Arthritis of subtalar joint complex
>
> *Pain behind heel*
> Haglund's deformity ("pump bumps," "heel bumps")
> Rupture of Achilles tendon
> Achilles paratendinitis
> Posterior tibial paratendinitis or tenosynovitis
> Peroneal paratendinitis or tenosynovitis
> Posterior calcaneal bursitis
> Calcaneal apophysitis
>
> *Pain beneath heel*
> Tender heel pad
> Plantar fasciitis

Sever's disease (calcaneal apophysitis)

This was thought to be an avascular necrosis of growing bone but is now interpreted as a chronic strain at the attachment of the posterior apophysis of the calcaneus to the main body of the bone, possibly from pull of the Achilles tendon. It is therefore analogous to Osgood-Schlatter disease of the tibial tuberosity.

Clinical features—The condition usually affects boys aged 8–13, who complain of a dull ache behind the heel of gradual onset that is exacerbated by jumping or just before heel lift. There is usually a limp with early heel lift. Rest normally relieves the pain. There is tenderness over the lower posterior part of the tuberosity of the calcaneus. Radiographs are usually normal.

Treatment—In most cases reassurance and advice about reducing activities will suffice: the condition usually subsides spontaneously. In some cases heel lifts help, and occasionally, if the pain is severe, a below knee walking cast is required.

Plantar calcaneal bursitis (policeman's heel)

This is inflammation of the adventitious bursa beneath the plantar aspect of the calcaneal tuberosities. It is associated with shearing stress due to an altered angle of heel strike.

Clinical features—Increasingly severe burning, aching, throbbing pain on the plantar surface of the heel. There is usually a history of increased activity or weight gain. The heel will seem normal but may feel warm. Direct pressure or sideways compression causes pain. The tissues may feel tight and congested.

Treatment—Rest and local anti-inflammatory drugs are useful. Heel cushions and medial arch supports may help, as may ultrasound treatment or shortwave diathermy.

Chronic inflammation of the heel pad

This is a distinct clinical condition that usually results from trauma or heavy heel strike. It is sometimes seen in elderly people as their fat pads atrophy or in those who suddenly become more active.

Clinical features—A generalised warm dull throbbing pain is felt over the weight bearing area of the heel, developing over a few months. The pain is typically most intense on first rising. There is tenderness over the heel, which feels tight and distended.

Treatment—Normally it improves with time and rest. Soft heel cushions and medial arch fillers sometimes help. Ultrasound treatment and short wave diathermy are often used, but controlled trials are few. Hydrocortisone injections are helpful only if very small areas of pain can be pinpointed. The injection can be more painful than the condition unless it is done carefully with adequate slow infiltration of local anaesthetic (or an ankle tibial nerve block) before injection of the corticosteroid.

Achilles tendon affections

Inflammation of the Achilles tendon and surrounding soft tissue may be associated with overuse or systemic inflammatory disorders. Inflammation of the tendon, peritendon tissues, and bursae provide slightly different clinical pictures. Conditions such as xanthoma can also affect the Achilles tendon, producing a fusiform swelling in the tendon. In such cases cholesterol concentrations should be checked and, if raised, treated.

Clinical features vary according to the tissues affected. Increased activity leading to an overuse syndrome may be a feature in younger active patients. Tendinitis presents as a painful local swelling of the tendon that moves with the tendon as the foot is dorsiflexed and plantar flexed. It is important to check the tendon for evidence of partial or complete rupture, which is often missed because of inflammation. Peritendinitis presents as a large diffuse swelling of the tissues surrounding the tendon that remains static as the tendon is stretched. Patients experience pain and crepitus on palpation. Achilles tendon bursitis presents as a diffuse fusiform swelling inferior to the Achilles tendon filling the normal indentation seen below the malleoli and deep to the Achilles tendon.

Treatment depends on the primary pathology. Partial or complete ruptures of the tendon require immobilisation and surgical repair. For inflammatory pathologies, non-steroidal anti-inflammatory drugs may help, as well as ultrasound treatment, friction, rest, and shock absorbing heel lifts. Sometimes inflammation may be triggered by overuse through poor foot mechanics; in such cases orthoses prescribed to control the pronation may help. Hydrocortisone injections may be useful if the bursa or peritendons are affected but are contraindicated for the tendon itself.

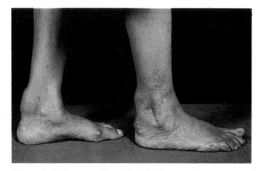

Chronic inflammation of Achilles tendon is another cause of heel pain. This should not be treated by local injection of corticosteroid.

Arthropathies affecting the foot

Common abnormalities in the rheumatoid foot

- Hallux valgus
- Lesser toe deformities—hammer toes, claw toes, etc
- Prominent metatarsal heads with overlying painful callosities or ulceration
- Pronation of foot with valgus heel deformity and collapse of mid-tarsal joint, giving a flatfooted appearance
- Tensynovitis, especially of the tibialis posterior and peroneal tendons, plantar heel bursitis, calcaneal spur, and tendoachilles bursitis
- Tarsal tunnel nerve compression syndrome

Osteoarthritis

Osteoarthritis in the foot may be asymptomatic but can lead to pain, joint stiffness, functional loss, and disability. The commonest sites are the first metatarso-phalangeal joint (hallux rigidus) and the tarsus joints. Biomechanical factors are often involved in the development of degenerative joint changes (for example, compensatory foot pronation in subtalar osteoarthritis). Trauma, recurrent urate gout, and the demands of fashion—such as inappropriate footwear—are other factors. However, the broad styles of modern shoes may actually be beneficial.

Pain in the foot

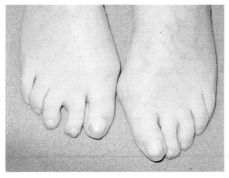

Metatarsal synovitis in early rheumatoid foot: note early hallux valgus of left foot and widening of second cleft of right foot—the "daylight sign."

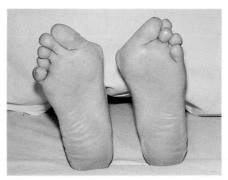

Plantar aspect of rheumatoid foot: note bilateral valgus drift and prominent metatarsal heads.

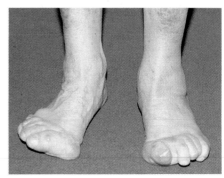

Advanced rheumatoid foot: note hind foot eversion, valgus clawing of toes, and pressure on metatarsal heads.

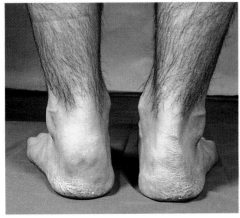

Ankylosing spondylitis of the feet: the hind foot is predominantly affected.

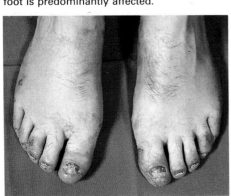

Psoriatic arthropathy.

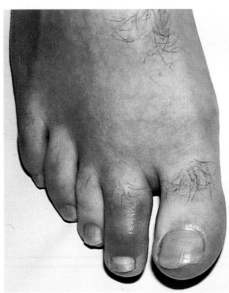

Reiter's syndrome—sausage toe (this is also found with psoriatic arthropathy).

Rheumatoid arthritis

Rheumatoid arthritis often starts in the foot, particularly at the metatarsophalangeal joints. The forefoot is painful and stiff; direct transverse pressure to the forefoot or squeezing a single metatarsophalangeal joint is painful. Non-specific metatarsalgia is often diagnosed. In the early stages of the disease, the hindfoot, particularly the subtalar joint, may also be painful. Synovitis of tendon sheaths around the ankle may also occur. In the chronic rheumatoid foot, severe pain in the forefoot may continue, with a sensation of walking on pebbles. Gross deformity causes dysfunction and disability.

Ankylosing spondylitis

Peripheral arthropathy of the feet is usually mild, but toe retraction, Achilles peritendinitis, and retrocalcaneal bursitis can be seen. In radiographs inflammatory spurs may be seen on the calcaneum at the insertion points of the Achilles tendon and plantar fascia.

Psoriatic arthritis

The pattern of articular involvement in the foot may vary from a single "sausage toe" (dactylitis) to a very destructive arthritis. Painful stiff interphalangeal and metatarsophalangeal joints, often in an asymmetrical pattern, are common. Claw toe and hallux valgus deformity are more obvious. Nail dystrophy may be seen, with typical pitting, onycholysis, subungual hyperkeratosis, discoloration, and transverse ridging. Pustular psoriasis on the plantar aspect of the foot may contribute to the pain experienced when walking. Asymmetrical heel pain may result from a plantar calcaneal enthesopathy.

Reiter's syndrome

Peripheral arthropathy, usually asymmetrical, associated with Reiter's syndrome is more common and more severe in the feet than the hands. Erosions can be seen in the proximal interphalangeal joints of the toes, the interphalangeal joint of the hallux, and the metatarsophalangeal joints. An early feature is pain in the plantar heel, the result of an enthesopathy at the ligament-bone junction of the plantar fascia and calcaneum. The typical skin lesion of Reiter's syndrome—keratoderma blenorrhagica—may be present on the soles of the feet.

Juvenile chronic arthritis

The knee and ankle joints are most often affected in all subtypes of juvenile chronic arthritis. Children may present with a limp or reluctance to walk. In the hind foot pain and reflex muscle spasm can lead to valgus deformity (in two thirds of cases) or varus deformity (in a third of cases). In some patients this may progress to bony ankylosis. There may be reluctance to push off with the forefoot during walking, and pressure studies reveal poor foot contact. Disuse can lead to delayed maturation of bone or soft tissue, and in such cases discrepancy in leg length should be carefully checked for.

Gout

The manifestations of acute gout in the foot are described in chapter 8. In the chronic state tophi in the foot may ulcerate if they act as pressure points. Permanent destructive joint damage and deformity may result and lead to painful dysfunction in the foot.

Management of rheumatic foot conditions

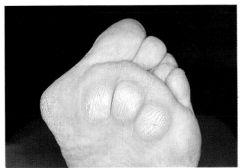

Metatarsophalangeal callosities in rheumatoid foot.

Patients with rheumatic foot problems are best managed by a team that includes a physician, a surgeon, and therapists. Podiatrists have a particular role in several aspects of care.

Tissue viability—Joint deformity causes pressure lesions such as callosities, corns, or ulceration and may be compounded by other factors such as ingrowing toe nails, peripheral neuropathy, or the effects of systemic corticosteroids. Podiatrists undertake procedures such as scalpel reduction, design and manufacture of insoles and orthoses, and surgery under local anaesthesia to relieve pain and restore or maintain tissue viability.

Foot function—Foot dysfunction due to arthritis can be improved with orthoses, either ready made or individually designed from casts. Orthoses may be used to control deformity—such as the valgus heel seen in rheumatoid arthritis—but also have a major role in maintaining tissue viability and relieving pain (be it joint, soft tissue, or skin lesion in origin).

Foot health promotion—Patients will often require advice on daily care of feet. Family members may be involved when patients cannot reach their feet or are unable to perform tasks to the feet because of other disability. Advice may be needed on splints, walking aids, footwear, insoles, foot hygiene, and exercise.

Foot surgery may be effective for relieving pain and improving deformity when conservative measures have failed. Many rheumatic patients have toe nail pathologies that require surgery under local anaesthetic, and those are best dealt with by an experienced clinician such as a podiatrist.

> The use of orthoses for rheumatic foot problems requires suitable footwear, and podiatrists should liaise with orthotists when extra depth shoes or surgical shoes are needed

6 FIBROMYALGIA SYNDROME

Michael Doherty, Adrian Jones

Fibromyalgia is common in hospital practice. It is rarely reported in children, and most patients are in their 40s or 50s. In all settings there is a strong female preponderance (about 90%). It is well reported in the United States, Canada, and Europe, but racial and social predisposition have not been adequately addressed.

Symptoms are variable. Pain and fatiguability are usually prominent and associated with considerable disability and handicap. Although patients can usually dress and wash independently, they cannot cope with a job or ordinary household activities. Pain is predominantly axial and diffuse but can affect any region and may at times be felt all over. Characteristically, analgesics, non-steroidal anti-inflammatory drugs, and local physical treatments are ineffective and may even worsen symptoms.

Patients often have a poor sleep pattern with considerable latency and frequent arousal. Typically they awake exhausted and feel more tired in the morning than later in the day. Unexplained headache, urinary frequency, and abdominal symptoms are common and may have been extensively investigated with no cause found. Patients usually score highly on measures of anxiety and depression.

Although the term fibromyalgia syndrome is not ideal, it does not imply causation and describes the commonest symptom. Idiopathic diffuse pain syndrome, generalised rheumatism, and non-restorative sleep disorder are terms that are increasingly preferred by some.

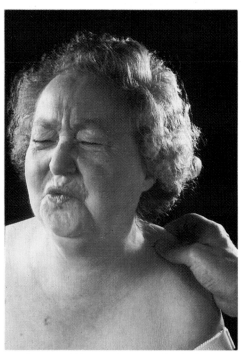

Typical hyperalgesic withdrawal response by patient with fibromyalgia. (Picture reproduced with patient's permission.)

Prevalence of fibromyalgia

Rheumatology clinics	20%
Internal medicine clinics	6%
Family practice clinics	2%
General medical inpatients	
United Kingdom	5%
General population	
Swedish city, British general practice	1%
American city	2%

Principal symptoms of fibromyalgia

Pain
Predominantly axial (neck and back), but may be all over
Often aggravated by stress, cold, and activity
Often associated with generalised morning stiffness
Often with subjective swelling of extremities
Paraesthesiae and dysaesthesiae of hands and feet

Fatiguability
Often extreme, occurring after minimal exertion

Non-restorative sleep
Waking unrefreshed
Poor concentration and forgetfulness
Low affect, irritable, and weepy

Headache
Occipital and bifrontal

Diffuse abdominal pain and variable bowel habit

Urinary frequency
Urgency (day and night)
Dysmenorrhoea

Clinical signs

Principal clinical findings

- Discordance between symptoms and disability and objective findings
- No objective weakness, synovitis, or neurological abnormality
- Multiple hyperalgesic tender sites (axial and upper and lower limbs)
- Pronounced tenderness to rolling of skin fold (mid-trapezius)
- Cutaneous hyperaemia after palpation of tender sites or rolling of skin fold
- Negative control (non-tender) sites (such as forehead, distal forearm, and lateral fibular head)

Clinical findings are unremarkable, and the principal positive sign is the presence of multiple hyperalgesic tender sites. In normal subjects these tender sites are uncomfortable to firm pressure, but in patients with fibromyalgia similar pressure produces a wince or withdrawal response. The degree of pressure is clearly important; delivery of standard pressure with a spring device (dolorimeter) is ideal, but reasonable palpation suffices for clinical purposes.

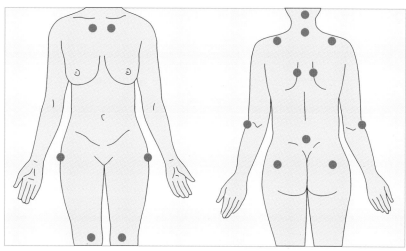

Common hyperalgesic tender sites.

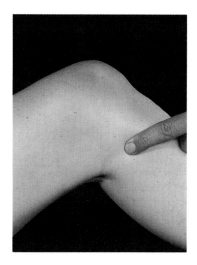
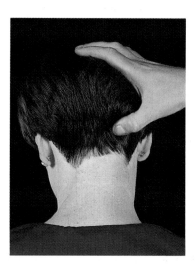

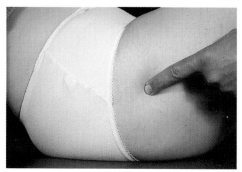

Palpation of hyperalgesic tender sites: (top left) medial fat pad of knee, (top right) site of muscle insertion at occiput, and (left) greater trochanter of femur.

Common hyperalgesic tender sites

- Low cervical spine (C4–C6 interspinous ligaments)
- Low lumbar spine (L4–S1 interspinous ligaments)
- Suboccipital muscle (posterior base of skull)
- Mid-supraspinatus
- Mid-point of upper trapezius
- Pectoralis insertion—maximal lateral to second costochondral junction
- Lateral epicondyle—tennis elbow sites, 1–2 cm distal to epicondyle
- Gluteus medius—upper, outer quadrant of buttock
- Greater trochanter
- Medial fat pad of knee

Hyperalgesia at one or two sites in the same quadrant often results from periarticular lesions or referred tenderness from an axial structure. In fibromyalgia, however, hyperalgesia is widespread and symmetrical. The number of tender sites required by different diagnostic criteria varies, but eight or more are sufficient for clinical purposes. Importantly, hyperalgesia is absent at sites that are normally non-tender. If a patient claims to be tender all over, fabrication or psychiatric disturbance (psychogenic rheumatism) is more likely. Osteoarthritis and periarticular syndromes are common and may be present as incidental findings or as a trigger for the syndrome.

Differential diagnosis

Differential diagnosis and investigations

Differential diagnosis	Investigations
Hypothyroidism	Thyroid function tests
Systemic lupus erythematosus	Full blood count
	Erythrocyte sedimentation rate and blood viscosity
	Antinuclear factor
Inflammatory myopathy	Creatine kinase concentration
Hyperparathyroidism	Calcium concentration and alkaline
Osteomalacia	phosphatase concentration

Other conditions that may present with widespread pain, weakness, or fatigue should be excluded by a limited investigational screen. Further tests may be warranted if a patient's history and examination suggest a predisposing or coexistent condition. Undertaking all investigations together reinforces the patient's confidence in the accuracy of the diagnosis and is preferable to a drawn out sequence of tests. Fibromyalgia may superimpose on pre-existing painful conditions such as osteoarthritis or cancer but usually affects subjects with no other diagnosis ("primary" fibromyalgia).

Nature of fibromyalgia

The pathogenesis of the syndrome remains unclear. Clinical heterogeneity is pronounced, and multiple factors are likely to relate to its development and chronicity. Depending on the predominant symptom, fibromyalgia may be categorised under various diagnostic labels. These conditions overlap and probably represent different expressions in a spectrum of abnormality. Medicine has a traditional bias towards a pathological explanation of disease, but with fibromyalgia there is no investigational evidence of overt inflammatory, metabolic, or structural abnormality and the problem appears functional rather than pathological.

Diagnostic terms that often include patients with fibromyalgia

Principal presenting symptom	Diagnostic label
Locomotor pain	Psychogenic rheumatism
	Fibrositis
	Pain amplification syndrome
Fatigue	Myalgic encephalomyelitis
	Chronic fatigue syndrome
Headache	Tension headache
Abdominal pain and bowel disturbance	Irritable bowel syndrome
Frequency and nocturia	Female urethral syndrome

Sleep disturbance

A strong association with sleep disturbance is suggested by:

- An increased frequency of non-restorative sleep

- Electroencephalographic evidence of reduced deep non-rapid eye movement (non-REM) sleep with interruption by α waves (α–δ intrusion)

- Reproduction of fibromyalgia symptoms and hyperalgesic tender sites in normal subjects by selective deprivation of non-REM (but not REM) sleep.

Chronic non-restorative sleep has been suggested as a possible cause. Various factors (such as regional pain syndrome, bereavement, and anxiety) cause reduced deep sleep, with resultant somatic symptoms and fatigue. Once reduced sleep has been established, reduced activity, declining aerobic fitness, and pain encourage perpetuation of this aberrant sleep pattern.

Possible mechanism of induction and perpetuation of fibromyalgia.

Other possible causes

Deficiency of serotonin (or its precursor tryptophan) and other abnormalities of the neuroendocrine axis have been proposed as mechanisms to explain both the sleep disorder and pain associated with fibromyalgia. Whether these reported abnormalities are cause or effect remains uncertain.

Whether the cause of fibromyalgia (such as signal misinterpretation, psychoneuroendocrine disorder, or aberrant pain mechanism) is peripheral or central remains unclear and may differ between patients

Viral aetiology has been proposed for patients with some forms of chronic fatigue syndrome, but evidence for triggering viral infections in most patients with fibromyalgia is lacking.

Affective symptoms are common, though whether they are primary or secondary remains unclear. In fibromyalgia the predominance of locomotor pain, presence of multiple hyperalgesic tender sites, development after selective sleep deprivation, and different response to treatment argue for differentiation from anxiety or depression with somatisation.

Management

There is no specific treatment for this condition, but individual patients may be considerably helped. The single most important intervention is a comprehensible explanation. Most patients expect a pessimistic cause for their devastating symptoms, and they should be reassured that the pain does not reflect cancer, inflammation, or structural damage. An explanation based on poor sleep and reduced fitness is readily understood and helps patients to rationalise their symptoms, disability, and treatments. It is helpful to include family members. Inquiry about life events may reveal problems that merit open discussion and counselling. Patients with sublimated anxiety are more likely to improve if their anxiety is identified and successfully addressed.

Controlled trials have confirmed the usefulness of low dose amitriptyline or dothiepin (25–75 mg at night) and a graded exercise programme to increase aerobic fitness.

Amitriptyline—The dose used is lower than that for depression. Its efficacy may be due to its normalising effects on the sleep centre or pain gating at the spinal cord level. Interestingly, cyclobenzaprine (a tricyclic muscle relaxant with no antidepressant action) is also effective. If these drugs are ineffective after a trial of four to six weeks, further drug treatment should be avoided. Benzodiazepines and other hypnotics have no place in treatment.

Increasing aerobic exercise is intended to improve sleep and restore fitness. It may initially exacerbate symptoms, but patients should be encouraged to continue despite pain (the opposite advice to that for someone with synovitis or joint damage). An important element is that the locus of control is now within the patient—it is up to them, not doctors or drugs, to improve their situation.

Operant and other illness behaviour is common. This needs to be recognised and eliminated by educating family members.

Coping strategies (such as meditational yoga) may permit patients to better control the extent to which pain and fatigue intervene in their life.

Prognosis

The prognosis for fibromyalgia is often poor. In one British study fewer than one in 10 patients diagnosed in hospital lost their symptoms over five years. Nevertheless, suitable advice can help most patients to learn to cope better with their condition and, importantly, to avoid further unnecessary investigations and drug treatments.

Principal strategies for managing fibromyalgia

- Educate patient
- Educate patient's family
- Avoid unnecessary investigations and treatments
- Use interventions to correct non-restorative sleep, improve aerobic fitness, and reinforce intrinsic locus of control

---

Interventions for managing fibromyalgia

Low dose amitriptyline
Initially a limited trial of 4–6 weeks

Graded aerobic exercise regimen
Individualised to patient
Set specified targets that increase weekly
Encourage small amounts often
Encourage continuation despite pain
Retrain to avoid operant behaviour

Coping strategies
Meditational yoga
Behavioural therapy

7 OSTEOARTHRITIS

Adrian Jones, Michael Doherty

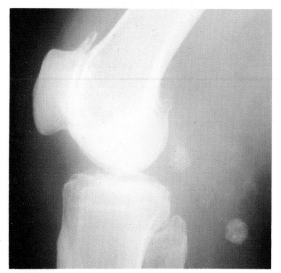

Radiograph of joint affected by osteoarthritis.

Osteoarthritis is the commonest condition to affect synovial joints, the single most important cause of locomotor disability, and a major challenge to health care. Previously considered as a degenerative disease that was an inevitable consequence of aging and trauma, osteoarthritis is now viewed as a metabolically dynamic, essentially reparative process that is increasingly amenable to treatment.

There is no generally accepted definition of osteoarthritis, but most would agree that pathologically it is a condition of synovial joints characterised by focal cartilage loss and an accompanying reparative bone response. Defining this in practice is less easy. Current definition of clinical cases hinges on detecting structural changes clinically or in radiographs. For many the plain radiograph remains the best means of assessment, with evidence of cartilage loss (joint space narrowing) and bone response (presence of osteophytes and sclerosis) being the main criteria. This definition, however, excludes joints with early minimal change, ignores tissues other than cartilage and bone, and omits consideration of biological consequences (symptoms and disability). There is often considerable discordance between structural change and clinical outcome; patients with apparent structural catastrophe may have few or no symptoms. Better understanding of the causes of symptoms and disability is currently a key challenge.

Process of osteoarthritis

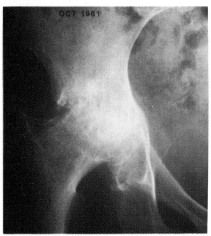

Example of healing osteoarthritis in hip joint.

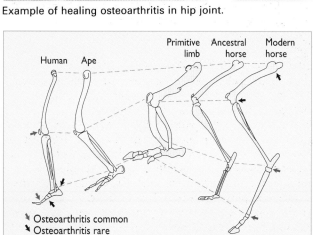

Association between osteoarthritis and evolution.

Observations about osteoarthritis have led to the suggestion that it is an aspect of the inherent repair process of synovial joints:
● Osteoarthritis has been present throughout evolution and is ubiquitous in humans and other vertebrates.
● Osteoarthritis is not simply the attrition of joint structures but is a metabolically active condition that shows a variable balance between anabolic and catabolic processes—at different stages there is increased activity in all joint tissues (cartilage, bone, synovium, capsule, and muscle)
● Osteoarthritis is common but is usually asymptomatic
● Occasionally, there is radiographic evidence of osteoarthritis joints "healing."

In most cases this slow but metabolically active process keeps pace with various triggering insults and is non-progressive, but sometimes it fails to compensate, resulting in joint failure (symptoms and disability). This interpretation partly explains the heterogeneity of osteoarthritis: various extrinsic and intrinsic insults cause different patterns of arthritis, and multiple constitutional and environmental factors modify response and outcome. Osteoarthritis targets specific joints, possibly those that have undergone recent evolutionary change in function (particularly relating to bipedal locomotion and precision grip) without yet adapting adequately.

Risk factors

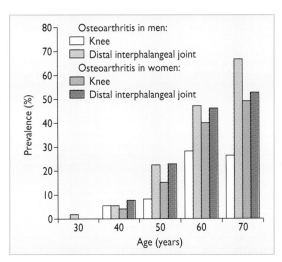

Prevalence of radiographic evidence of osteoarthritis in the population.

Age

Although not an inevitable consequence of aging, osteoarthritis is strongly related to age. This may represent cumulative insult to the joint, possibly aggravated by decline in neuromuscular function, or senescence of homoeostatic repair mechanisms. The consequence is a considerable medical burden and one that will increase with increasing numbers of elderly people in the British population. In general:

● Osteoarthritis is uncommon (and multiple joint osteoarthritis is rare) in people aged under 45
● Prevalence of osteoarthritis increases up to age 65, when at least half of people have radiographic evidence of osteoarthritis in at least one joint group
● Prevalence of symptomatic osteoarthritis also increases with age, but data for this association are less clear (for example, the knee is affected in about 15% of people aged over 55)
● Increases in prevalence (symptomatic and asymptomatic osteoarthritis) over the age of 65 are less clear.

Sex

There is a pronounced female preponderance for severe radiographic grades of osteoarthritis, osteoarthritis of the hand and knee, and symptoms.

Ethnic groups

Osteoarthritis of the hip is uncommon in black and Asian populations compared with white people, and polyarticular osteoarthritis of the hand is rare in black Africans and Malaysians. This difference seems to reflect genetic rather than cultural differences.

Individual risk factors

There are two main categories of such risk factors: generalised factors (such as obesity, genetic factors, and being female) and localised factors resulting in abnormal mechanical loading at specific sites (such as meniscectomy, instability, and dysplasia). An inherited defect in type II collagen has been described in a rare familial condition of polyarticular osteoarthritis of premature onset, but the genetics of common osteoarthritis is unknown. Some factors (such as obesity, muscle function, and occupation) may be modified and thus offer scope for primary, secondary, and tertiary prevention.

Putative risk factors for development and progression of hip and knee osteoarthritis

Hip	Knee
Development	
Previous disease or trauma (such as Perthes' disease or slipped femoral epiphysis)	Previous trauma (such as meniscectomy)
Acetabular dysplasia	Distal femoral dysplasia
Avascular necrosis	Medial femoral necrosis
Non-gonococcal septic arthritis	Non-gonococcal septic arthritis
Occupation (farming)	Sex (female)
Progression	
Superior pole pattern	Pronounced varus
Chondrocalcinosis (knee)	Sex (female)
Obesity	Obesity
Use of non-steroidal anti-inflammatory drugs	Use of non-steroidal anti-inflammatory drugs
"Protective" factors	
Osteoporosis	

Types of osteoarthritis

Despite attempts to subdivide osteoarthritis according to various criteria, there are no sharp divisions in the spectrum of osteoarthritis. People may display different features at different sites and evolve from one "subset" to another. Nevertheless certain distinctions may be useful.

Nodal generalised osteoarthritis (menopausal osteoarthritis)

This common condition is clustered in families and is characterised by multiple Heberden's nodes (distal interphalangeal joint) and Bouchard's nodes (proximal interphalangeal joint); symptoms commonly starting around the menopause; polyarticular osteoarthritis of the interphalangeal joints; and later development of osteoarthritis of the knee, hip, and apophyseal joint. Its outcome, particularly with respect to hand symptoms and function, is generally good. Its aetiology is unknown, but the reported association with the HLA A1B8 gene, the occurrence of immune complexes in affected joint tissues, and the high prevalence (50%) of seropositivity for IgG rheumatoid factor supports the idea of a single immune mediated insult in genetically predisposed subjects.

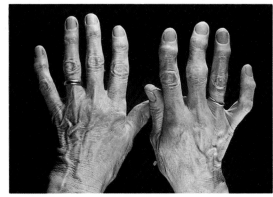

Nodal osteoarthritis.

Osteoarthritis

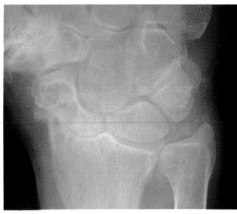

Radiograph of wrist showing chondrocalcinosis and arthropathy.

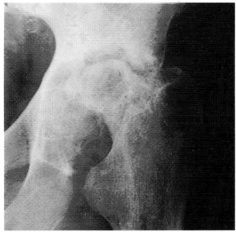

Apatite associated destructive arthritis of hip.

Crystal associated osteoarthritis

Calcium crystals, notably calcium pyrophosphate dihydrate and apatite, may deposit in cartilage as an isolated phenomenon but also commonly occur in osteoarthritic joints. In this context they probably arise via physicochemical changes accompanying the osteoarthritis process. Although these crystals may sometimes initiate inflammation (such as in acute pseudogout), they usually have no direct deleterious effects.

Osteoarthritis with deposition of calcium pyrophosphate dihydrate (pyrophosphate arthropathy) occurs predominantly in elderly women, principally affects the knee, and is associated with inflammation and widespread and pronounced radiographic changes (usually hypertrophic).

Apatite associated destructive arthritis—Although modest amounts of apatite are present in most osteoarthritic joints, large amounts occur in apatite associated destructive arthritis. This is almost totally confined to the hips, shoulders (Milwaukee shoulder), and knees of elderly women and has a poor outcome. There is typically rapid painful progression with large cool effusions, progressive instability, and atrophic radiographic changes. The differential diagnosis includes Charcot arthropathy, sepsis, and avascular necrosis.

Osteoarthritis of premature onset

Development of single joint osteoarthritis after severe trauma or alteration in joint biomechanics (for example, after meniscectomy or because of developmental abnormality) is not uncommon. However, premature onset (under the age of 50) in several joints should prompt consideration of prediposing metabolic, hormonal, or other causes. Conditions for which such osteoarthritis can be the presenting feature are rare, but some are amenable to correction (although existing osteoarthritis is usually unaffected). These conditions include:

- Haemochromatosis
- Ochronosis
- Acromegaly
- Spondyloepiphyseal dysplasia, epiphyseal dysplasia, and hereditary type II collagen defects
- Thiemann's disease
- Endemic osteoarthritis (normally rare but common in endemic areas).

Clinical features

The main clinical features of osteoarthritis are symptoms, functional impairment, and signs. There can be considerable discordance between these three. Pain may arise from several sites in and around an osteoarthritic joint. Suggested mechanisms include increased capsular and intraosseous pressure, subchondral microfracture, and enthesopathy or bursitis secondary to muscle weakness and structural alteration. Severity of pain and functional impairment are greatly influenced by personality, anxiety, depression, and daily activity.

Crepitus, bony enlargement, deformity, instability, and restricted movement may occur in any combination and predominantly reflect structural change. Varying degrees of synovitis (warmth, effusion, and synovial thickening) may be superimposed, and muscle weakness or wasting is usual. Periarticular sources of pain are often found, particularly at the knee and hip.

Assessment is directed at establishing the sources of symptoms in an individual patient. Determining the presence of osteoarthritis is not usually the problem—the usual question is whether osteoarthritis is relevant to the patient's complaints. The high prevalance of osteoarthritis in the general population means that comorbid conditions often exist. These include soft tissue lesions (enthesopathy and bursitis), fibromyalgia, gout, inflammatory arthritis, and sepsis. These require attention in their own right. Only an adequate history and examination can determine how much structural and inflammatory change is present and how much this contributes to a patient's overall problem.

Treatment

The aims of treatment are patient education, pain relief, optimisation of function, and minimisation of progression.

Changes in lifestyle for patients with osteoarthritis

General measures
Maintain optimal weight
Encourage activity and regular general exercise
Maintain positive approach

Specific measures
Strengthening of local muscles
Use of appropriate footwear and walking aids
Pay attention to specific problems caused by disability (such as shopping, housework, and job)

Drug treatments for osteoarthritis

Adequate doses of simple analgesics
Topical preparations (non-steroidal anti-inflammatory drugs and rubefacients)
Non-steroidal anti-inflammatory drugs—only for patients whose symptoms are not controlled by other means or during acute exacerbations; regularly review their continued use
Intra-articular corticosteroid injections—consider for patients who are unfit for surgery or for acute flares

Surgical treatments for osteoarthritis

History of joint locking—consider arthroscopy for removal of loose body
Persistent synovitis—consider arthroscopic washout or radioisotope synovectomy
Joint replacement is highly effective for hip and knee—consider early referral for opinion

Biomechanical factors

Weight reduction is desirable in obese patients and may reduce progression of knee osteoarthritis. Muscle strength is associated with disability. Increasing strength and aerobic fitness is possible in all age groups and is beneficial to osteoarthritic joints and personal wellbeing. Insoles to counteract knee varus deformity, patellofemoral strapping, walking sticks, and cushioned shoes (trainers) are useful in redistributing stress and reducing impact loading.

Pain control

Pain is the main reason why patients seek help. The current high use of non-steroidal anti-inflammatory drugs for osteoarthritis is probably mistaken. Adequate doses of analgesics such as paracetamol given regularly are usually adequate for most patients. Symptoms of osteoarthritis are often episodic, and if non-steroidal anti-inflammatory drugs are used their requirement should be regularly re-evaluated, especially in elderly patients who are at risk. There is as yet no convincing evidence that these drugs affect progression of osteoarthritis in humans, but hastening of progression (especially by indomethacin) has been suggested.

Topical non-steroidal anti-inflammatory drugs have similar efficacy to oral preparations in patients with osteoarthritis, but since they have fewer side effects they probably should be used more often, particularly for patients with just a few symptomatic, readily accessible joints. However, there remains substantial doubt as to their superiority over simple rubefacients. Several other symptomatic treatments (some with claimed chondroprotective action) are available in some countries or are under investigation. There is considerable interest in pharmacological manipulation of osteoarthritis (and exciting experimental data), but the precise role of such drugs in treatment is not yet defined.

Disease modifying drugs

The use of intra-articular corticosteroid injections for uncomplicated osteoarthritis is controversial and generally not recommended. They have a place, however, in treating patients with acute crystal associated synovitis or those who are unfit for or awaiting surgery. Their effect is generally transient. Similarly, the place of radioisotope synovectomy is unclear, although injections of yttrium-90 may benefit some patients with osteoarthritis and persistent synovitis of large joints.

Surgery

The success of prosthetic joint replacements has greatly advanced management of end stage hip and knee osteoarthritis. Although issues relating to funding, waiting times, choice of prosthesis, and revision have to be faced, there is no doubt that such surgery can transform patients' lives. Other surgical approaches (arthroscopic lavage, osteotomy, and arthrodesis) may also be useful. The criteria for surgery are not definite but should probably include uncontrolled pain (particularly nocturnal pain) and severe impairment of function. Age, in itself, is not a contraindication.

Psychological factors

A major contribution to managing osteoarthritis has been the demonstration that a patient's psychological status (anxiety, depression, and social support) is an important determinant of symptomatic and functional outcome. Providing social support, even just regular telephone contact with a lay person, can effectively ameliorate symptoms. Perhaps the single most important help that any therapist can give is to emphasise to patients that osteoarthritis is not invariably progressive, that things can be done, and that the patients are not on their own.

The authors thank the Arthritis and Rheumatism Council, United Kingdom, for financial support.

8 GOUT, HYPERURICAEMIA, AND CRYSTAL ARTHRITIS

Michael L Snaith

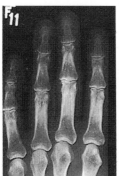

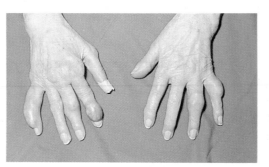

Chronic, relatively painless, tophaceous gouty arthritis of fingers, probably due to patient's long term treatment with diuretics.

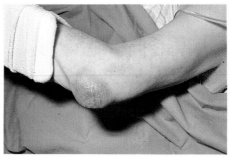

Acute gouty olecranon bursa. This, the patient's first attack of gout for many years, occurred after major bowel surgery.

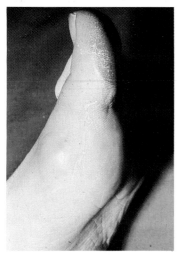

Classic podagra: acute gouty arthritis of first metatarsophalangeal joint.

The term gout is sometimes loosely used to describe an acutely painful foot, but it is best reserved for those cases where deposition of crystals of uric acid (urate) is thought to be the cause of pain. The big toe (first metatarsophalangeal) joint is the classic site for urate gout, and an overweight, overindulgent man is the traditional sufferer. However, a substantial minority of patients (perhaps 30%) first get their gout at another site (such as other parts of the foot, the knee, the hand, or the shoulder), and, with more older women in the population and the widespread use of diuretics (which raise blood urate concentrations), this traditional view needs revising.

Gout is a condition of occasional attacks and long periods of remission. The prevalence of people at risk is therefore quite different from the incidence of actual attacks: a general practice with a list of 2000 patients might have 15 men and 3 women with a tendency to gout. Although most such patients are managed in primary care, acute gout may be precipitated by diuretics or by stresses such as acute infection, ketosis, or surgery, and cases therefore also crop up in hospital.

Chronic gouty arthritis is not common but can still be found, even though in most cases it can be treated and prevented. The x ray appearance is characteristic and should not be confused with other forms of arthritis. Tophi develop mainly in the ear but also occur elsewhere.

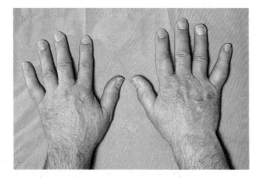

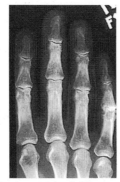

Hands of patient with chronic gouty arthritis (top) and his radiographs (bottom). Note lack of perarticular osteopenia and that the punched out erosions, especially at the right little finger proximal interphalangeal joint, are a little further away from joint margin than would be found with rheumatoid arthritis.

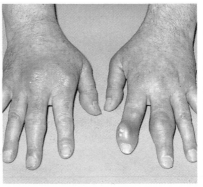

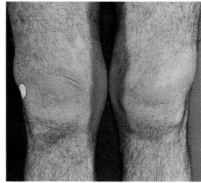

Chronic gouty arthritis may come to resemble other forms of inflammatory synovitis, such as here, with dorsal swelling of the wrist (left) and bilateral large knee effusions (right), from which urate crystals were identified. The arthritis resolved on appropriate treatment.

Acute gout

The most important differential
diagnosis for acute gout is infection

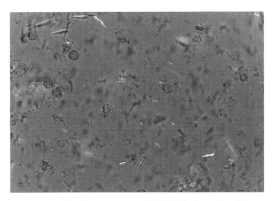

Urate crystals from synovial fluid viewed with
compensated polarised light: about the same length
as the diameter of a polymorphonuclear leucocyte
and negatively birefringent (coloured yellow when
aligned parallel to axis of slow vibration of the red
compensator inserted between polariser and
analyser, and coloured blue when not so aligned).

Treatment of acute gout

Non-steroidal anti-inflammatory drugs *or*
Colchicine
Avoid aspirin
Do not treat with allopurinol or uricosuric
  drugs

Diagnosis

Few things are as painful as a severe attack of gout: it often develops overnight and reaches a peak within hours so that, with an affected foot, it is impossible to bear weight or even the touch of bedclothes. The skin is red and may peel; nothing else except infection causes this, so infection is the most important differential diagnosis. Left to itself (which it rarely is) acute gout will start to improve in a week or two but will not settle completely for about a month.

A slight fever, leucocytosis, raised erythrocyte sedimentation rate and plasma viscosity, and increased C reactive protein concentration are all non-specific indicators of inflammation and will be variably abnormal depending on the severity of gout. Blood urate concentration cannot be relied on to confirm or exclude gout: in a small proportion of cases it is normal during an attack but raised at other times. If it is feasible, fresh synovial fluid or tissue should be examined under polarised light for the presence of urate crystals, which can usually be clearly distinguished from pyrophosphate crystals of pseudogout.

Management

Non-steroidal anti-inflammatory drugs are much more effective for acute gout than any analgesic. A history of peptic ulcer is a relative contraindication, but appropriate H_2 blockade should permit treatment with non-steroidal anti-inflammatory drugs in most cases. There is no clear advantage in any one preparation, but a large dose of naproxen (1·5 g) or indomethacin (150 mg) on the first day, being reduced thereafter, is known to be effective. When non-steroidal anti-inflammatory drugs are clearly contraindicated colchicine is useful; 0·5 mg taken orally every three hours for 12 hours, with the dose being reduced thereafter. Diarrhoea is a probable side effect, but this soon settles after withdrawal of the drug. If all else fails, an intramuscular injection of a corticosteroid, such as 40 mg of methylprednisolone, is effective treatment for acute gout.

Gout is associated with hypertension and heart disease, and a patient's visit to general practice after an attack provides a good opportunity to practise preventive medicine.

Hyperuricaemia

Causes of hyperuricaemia

Endogenous	*Exogenous*
Family history	Dietary purines
Body build	Alcohol
Cell breakdown	Drugs
Renal function	
Hypertension	

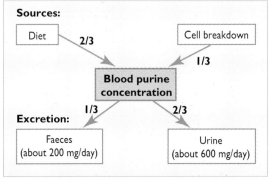

Outline of purine metabolism.

The risk of developing gout increases with increasing hyperuricaemia, but the rise is not proportional and there is no point at which gout is inevitable. Many factors are associated with a raised urate concentration. With normal renal function and an absence of drugs that affect renal handling of urate, its blood concentration depends mainly on the breakdown of nuclear proteins from internal catabolism and external purine load. Genetic factors are also important, but, apart from rare inborn errors of metabolism, the inheritance is polygenic.

The upper normal limit for serum or plasma urate concentration is about 420 µmol/l (7 mg/100 ml) in adult men and postmenopausal women and 360 µmol/l (6 mg/100 ml) in premenopausal women. The risk of gout rises appreciably with concentrations over 600 µmol/l. There is a small diurnal variation in blood concentration. A low purine diet can reduce blood concentrations of urate by up to 15% and urinary excretion by rather more, so attention to diet in patients with habitually high intakes of purine can significantly reduce risk. Faecal urate is not an important consideration in diagnosis or management.

Management of hyperuricaemia and a tendency to gout

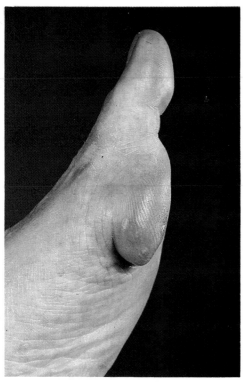

Tophus on foot of a man whose chronic gout had been treated with allopurinol 300 mg daily for many years. This diminished after adoption of a strict diet.

In an otherwise healthy person, the likeliest risk of a raised urate concentration is gout; formation of kidney stones and renal damage depend on other factors, so isolated hyperuricaemia should not normally be treated with allopurinol. The exceptions are the use of prophylactic allopurinol to prevent acute renal failure in patients given cytotoxic drugs or radiotherapy, and occasionally to treat a highly hyperuricaemic patient with an increased risk of stones who may become dehydrated.

There are various options for managing hyperuricaemia, and most patients usually have a preference once the risks have been explained.

Treating occasional acute attacks of gout

Some hyperuricaemic patients may suffer an acute attack as infrequently as once a year. They may be prepared to accept this risk and simply seek treatment for an attack as and when it occurs.

Reduction of risk by dieting

If dietary risk factors can be identified most patients prefer reducing these to a lifetime of taking pills. Crash diets for extremely obese patients are inappropriate: ketosis raises urate concentration and can cause an acute attack. A low purine diet consists of avoiding foods with high concentrations of metabolically active tissues. Examples are liver, kidneys, red meat, small muscular fish such as sardines, and vegetables such as pulses and whole grain cereals. Beer, lager, port, and some wines should be avoided: apart from their calorific value, they contain purines and the alcohol raises the blood lactate concentration.

Avoidance of drugs that affect urate excretion

Such drugs include aspirin in low doses and the second line antituberculous drug pyrazinamide, but thiazide diuretics are the likeliest to be encountered. There is no way of avoiding the risk if this group of drugs is necessary, and no thiazide is free of the effect.

Long term reduction in blood urate concentration

The two main choices of treatment are uricosuric drugs and allopurinol. In addition, the non-steroidal anti-inflammatory drugs azapropazone and tiaprofenic acid have a uricosuric effect and so have a place in the long term management of gout as well as acute treatment.

Uricosuric drugs—Probenecid (500 mg rising to 1500 mg a day) and sulphinpyrazone (100 mg rising to 600 mg a day) increase urate excretion and so are relatively contraindicated for patients with renal failure and absolutely so in patients with urate stones. Gastric intolerance is a relatively common problem with both drugs.

Allpurinol inhibits xanthine oxidase, diverting purine breakdown to xanthines, which are more soluble than urate. A dose of 100 mg a day, rising progressively to 300 mg a day, controls most cases of gout and eventually eliminates tophi, but doses of 600 mg a day or more are occasionally required.

A new attack of acute gout should never be treated with allopurinol or a uricosuric drug as these will prolong the attack (presumably because of a gradient between blood and tissue stores). Likewise, when the attack has settled the start of treatment should be accompanied by either colchicine (0·5 mg twice or thrice daily) or by a maintenance dose of a non-steroidal anti-inflammatory drug for at least four months. Even then sporadic attacks may occur for the first year of treatment.

Uricosuric drugs

Action
Reduce blood urate concentration and increase urine concentration of urate

Side effects
Mainly gastrointestinal intolerance

Contraindications
Presence of kidney stones
Acute gout

Concurrent treatment
Low dose of non-steroidal anti-inflammatory drug or colchicine for at least four months

---

Allopurinol

Action
Reduces blood and urine concentrations of urate

Side effects
Occasionally rashes or hepatitis

Contraindications
Acute gout

Concurrent treatment
Low dose of non-steroidal anti-inflammatory drug or colchicine for at least four months

Kidney and gout

Chronic lead poisoning from vessels
used to distil "moonshine" is still a cause
of gout and renal disease in some parts
of the world

Blood urate concentration does not rise until the glomerular filtration rate (creatinine clearance) falls to below about 20 ml a minute. People rarely get clinically important renal impairment from hyperuricaemia alone. Thus, although renal failure can occasionally present with gout and a patient may present with a first attack of gout and simultaneously be found to have renal impairment, a moderately raised concentration of urea or creatinine in the blood is unlikely to be the sole explanation of a raised blood urate concentration. Patients with chronic severe gout and tophi are more likely to have hyperuricosuria and stones, but they represent a small minority.

Patients who habitually form non-urate kidney stones may benefit from allopurinol, even if they have a normal urate concentration, as this drug seems to reduce urolithiasis in general. The association between hypertension and gout is obviously relevant to renal impairment.

Pseudogout and calcium pyrophosphate deposition disease

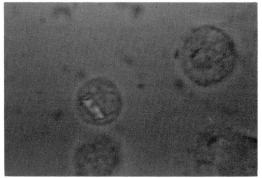

Crystals of calcium pyrophosphate viewed under compensated polarised light: crystals are usually short and stubby, often much smaller than urate crystals, and are weakly positively birefringent (blue when aligned with slow axis and yellow—as here—when perpendicular).

Pseudogout is an acute attack of inflammatory arthritis due to shedding of pyrophosphate crystals from articular cartilage. Chondrocalcinosis (radiological calcification of articular cartilage) is an essential prerequisite of the condition but is only strong circumstantial evidence in diagnosis. Confirmation requires the demonstration of crystals 1–10 µm long, rhomboidal, with weak positive birefringence (blue when aligned to the slow axis of the red compensator).

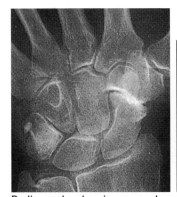
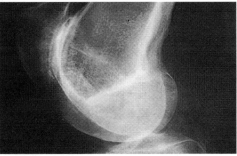

Radiographs showing examples of pyrophosphate arthritis: (left) calcified triangular ligament of wrist and (right) linear calcification at knee.

It is of a broadly similar nature to urate gout, but the affected joints are more likely to be the knee, wrist, or shoulder. Attacks are rarely quite as acute or severe as with urate gout but may be more difficult to diagnose: the patient may present with systemic features of fever and malaise sufficient to suspect sepsis, and crystals are often difficult to find in the synovial fluid, which should be centrifuged before examination. With other types of calcium pyrophosphate deposition disease, the arthritis may be more chronic and resemble non-erosive inflammatory arthritis, or the clinical picture may be that of osteoarthritis with episodes of inflammation and somewhat atypical joint pattern (wrists and shoulders, more genu valgus than genu varus).

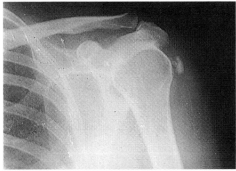

Radiograph showing calcification at insertion of rotator cuff.

Other forms of crystal arthropathy include post-traumatic or heterotopic calcium phosphate, calcific bursitis or periarthritis due to hydroxyapatite, and a rare destructive arthritis (Milwaukee syndrome) due to mixed crystal deposition. These conditions emphasise the need for a high quality analysis of synovial fluid to be available. This service should be in the pathology laboratory of hospitals and therefore accessible to all clinical departments rather than confined to interested rheumatologists or orthopaedic surgeons.

9 OSTEOPOROSIS

Nicola Peel, Richard Eastell

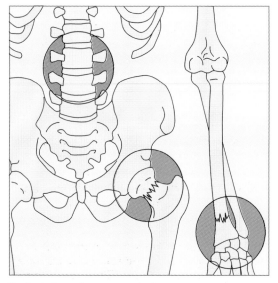

Typical sites of osteoporotic fracture.

Osteoporosis causes considerable morbidity and mortality, and there is evidence that the burden of this condition is increasing out of proportion to the changing demographic structure of populations in Western countries.

Osteoporosis may be defined as a disorder resulting from the combination of low bone mass (osteopenia) and low trauma fractures. Typical sites of osteoporotic fracture are the vertebral body, distal forearm, and proximal femur.

It is now possible to accurately determine individuals' risk of osteoporosis and to monitor their response to treatment by means of bone densitometry. Many cases of osteoporosis are preventable, and treatments are effective in reducing the number of further fractures in patients with established disease.

Pathophysiology

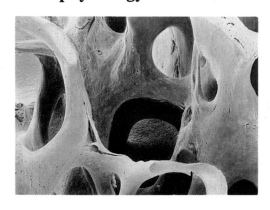

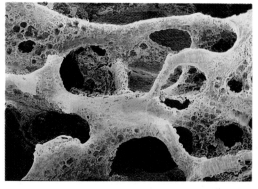

False colour, scanning electron micrographs of normal trabecular bone (left) and trabecular bone affected by osteoporosis (right).

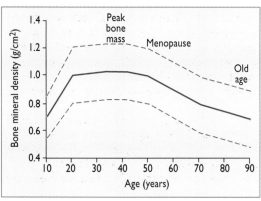

Association between age and bone mineral density of lumbar spine in women. (Lines show mean (2 SD)).

The human skeleton is composed of about 20% trabecular bone and 80% cortical bone. Bone undergoes a continual process of resorption and formation in discrete bone remodelling units. About 10% of the adult skeleton is remodelled each year. This turnover prevents fatigue damage and is important in maintaining calcium homoeostasis. Bone loss results from an imbalance between the rates of resorption and formation. Trabecular bone is more metabolically active, and osteoporotic fractures tend to occur at sites composed of more than 50% trabecular bone.

Bone loss leads to thinning, and in some cases perforation, of the trabecular plates. Trabecular perforation occurs in situations of increased bone turnover, and the resulting loss of normal architecture leads to a disproportionate loss of strength for the amount of bone lost.

- Peak bone mass is achieved by age 30.
- After skeletal maturity, bone is lost in both sexes at about 1% a year.
- Women experience a phase of accelerated bone loss for five to 10 years after the menopause.

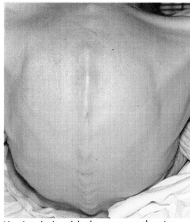

Kyphosis in elderly woman due to osteoporosis.

Clinical consequence of osteoporosis

Increased mortality—Mortality is increased by 20% in the first year after a hip fracture. It is also increased after vertebral fracture, possibly due to coexisting disease.

Pain usually occurs in the early stages of a fracture. Prolonged pain may be due to the development of secondary osteoarthritis. Pain can also result from the costal margin impinging on the pelvic brim.

Deformities include kyphosis, loss of height, and abdominal protrusion.

Loss of independence has a considerable financial impact since it may require long term community support or care in nursing homes after a hip fracture.

Epidemiology

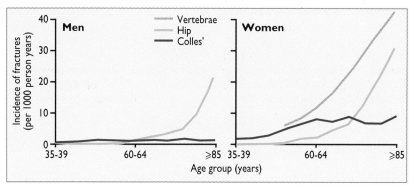

Incidence of osteoporotic fractures with age.

● One in two women and one is six men are likely to sustain an osteoporosis related fracture by the age of 90.

● The incidence of osteoporotic fractures is increasing more than would be expected from the aging of the population. This may reflect changing patterns of exercise or diet in recent decades.

Classification of osteoporosis

Primary
● Type I (postmenopausal)
● Type II (senile)
● Idiopathic (at ages <50)

Secondary
● Endocrine—Thyrotoxicosis, primary hyperparathyroidism, Cushing's syndrome, hypogonadism
● Gastrointestinal—Malabsorption syndrome (such as coeliac disease), partial gastrectomy, liver disease (such as primary biliary cirrhosis)
● Rheumatological—Rheumatoid arthritis, ankylosing spondylitis
● Malignancy—Multiple myeloma, metastatic carcinoma
● Drugs—Corticosteroids, heparin

Risk factors for osteoporosis

● Being female
● Being elderly
● Early menopause (age <45)
● Hypogonadism
● Smoking
● High alcohol intake
● Physical inactivity
● Thin body type
● Heredity

Classification of osteoporosis

Type I osteoporosis results from accelerated bone loss, probably as a result of oestrogen deficiency. The increased rate of bone loss leads to predominant loss of trabecular bone and frequent trabecular perforation. This typically results in fractures of vertebral bodies and of the distal forearm in women in their 60s and 70s.

Type II osteoporosis results from the slower age related bone loss that occurs in both sexes. There is less inequality between the rates of cortical and trabecular bone loss, and the typical manifestation is of fracture of the proximal femur in elderly people.

Secondary osteoporosis accounts for about 20% of cases in women and 40% of cases in men.

Risk factors

As well as being female and elderly, there are several well established risk factors for osteoporosis in populations. These risk factors do not, however, have adequate sensitivity or specificity to identify individuals at risk, and measurement of bone mineral density is necessary to predict a person's current and future risk of bone fracture.

Hypogonadism may be secondary to anorexia nervosa or excessive exercise.

Smoking—This effect may be mediated by smokers' tendency to have lower body weight and to have an earlier menopause than non-smokers.

High alcohol consumption may have a direct suppressive effect on bone formation and may also lead to hypogonadism. Weekly alcohol consumption of more than 14 units for women or 21 units for men may be toxic to bone.

Thin body type increases risk because conversion of androstenedione to oestrone occurs in adipose tissue in postmenopausal women.

Heredity—Genetic factors probably account for up to 70% of the variability in peak bone mass.

Investigations

Investigations for osteoporosis

Spinal radiographs
Bone densitometry
Screen for secondary causes
- Serum calcium, phosphate, alkaline phosphatase, and creatinine concentrations
- 24 Hour urinary calcium and creatinine excretion
- Serum protein electrophoresis
- Urinary Bence Jones protein concentration
- Thyroid stimulating hormone concentration
- Serum testosterone concentration (in men)

People with an osteoporosis related fracture should be investigated as shown. Those thought to be at risk of osteopenia should have a bone density measurement followed by further investigation if this confirms clinically important osteopenia.

Spinal radiographs

Up to half of vertebral fractures are asymptomatic. Radiographs of both the thoracic and lumbar spine are therefore necessary to detect existing fractures. However, osteopenia cannot be reliably diagnosed from the radiographic appearance, and bone densitometry is needed to quantify osteoporosis and to monitor the progression of the disease and response to treatment.

Bone densitometry

Bone density is usually measured by dual energy x ray absorptiometry, a technique that uses extremely low doses of ionising radiation to accurately and precisely quantify bone mineral density. Measurements are usually made of the lumbar spine and proximal femur, as these are the areas where osteoporotic fractures have the greatest clinical and financial impact.

Bone density is the main determinant of a person's risk of fracture. The predictive value of bone density is similar to that of blood pressure in determining the risk of cerebrovascular accident or of serum cholesterol for risk of coronary thrombosis. The relative risk of fracture increases two to three times for each standard deviation decrease in bone density. At low bone mineral density a small change in density results in a large change of risk of fracture. This has important implications for preventing and treating osteoporosis.

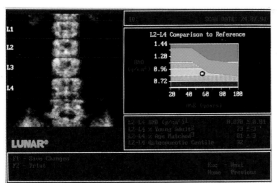

Bone density scan of lumbar spine

Indications for measuring bone density

Definite indications

Oestrogen deficiency—Particularly after early menopause or to help when considering hormone replacement therapy

Vertebral deformity or radiographic evidence of osteopenia— Asymptomatic vertebral deformity may be result of old trauma or represent Scheuermann's disease

Monitoring response of osteoporosis to treatment

Possible indications

Asymptomatic primary hyperparathyroidism— Parathyroidectomy may significantly increase bone mass

Screening for osteoporosis—Present evidence is insufficient to support introduction of widespread screening

Identifying patients with fast bone loss—Such patients are likely to show best response to antiresorptive therapy

Long term glucocorticoid treatment—Doses of >5 mg daily are thought to be deleterious to bone

Other forms of secondary osteoporosis

Treatment and prevention

Drugs to improve bone mass in osteopenic patients

Antiresorptive action

Hormone replacement therapy—Also helps in treating menopausal symptoms and preventing cardiovascular morbidity; treatment for at least five years is necessary for benefit; prolonged use (>10 years) may slightly increase risk of breast cancer

Cyclical disodium etidronate with calcium carbonate (Didronel PMO)—Poor absorption means that etidronate must be taken on an empty stomach

Calcitonin—Currently available as subcutaneous injection; a nasal preparation, claimed to have better tolerance, is being developed

Calcium (1000 mg daily)—Probably ineffective in perimenopausal women but seems useful in some older patients; has excellent safety profile

Vitamin D and calcium—Recent evidence suggests that this is useful for elderly patients; toxicity prevented by physiological doses of vitamin D

Anabolic steroids—Androgenic side effects make these drugs unacceptable for most women

Formation stimulating action

Fluoride—Dramatically increases bone mass, but evidence of preventing fractures is inconclusive; therapeutic window is probably narrow

---

Treating established osteoporosis

The aim of treating established osteoporosis is to alleviate patients' symptoms and to reduce the risk of further fractures. Currently available drugs are used to prevent further bone loss, and they can reduce the risk of further fractures by up to 50%.

Pain relief is provided mainly by analgesic drugs, but physical measures—such as lumbar support for a limited time or a transcutaneous nerve stimulator—are also useful. The pain from a fracture usually resolves within six months, but patients with vertebral fractures may require long term analgesia because of secondary degenerative disease.

Drugs to improve bone mass may act by inhibiting resorption of bone or by stimulating formation of bone.

Treating secondary causes often leads to partial recovery of bone mass.

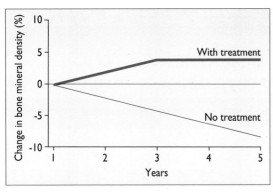

Probable effect of antiresorptive treatment on bone density in a patient losing 2% bone mass a year. After five years, treatment results in a net gain of 14% of untreated bone mass.

Prevention of osteoporosis

Optimising peak bone mass
- Exercise—Must be regular and weight bearing (such as walking or aerobics); excessive exercise may lead to bone loss
- Dietary calcium—May be important, especially during growth

Reducing rate of bone loss
- Hormone replacement therapy
- Regular exercise
- Maintain calcium intake
- Moderate alcohol intake
- Stop smoking

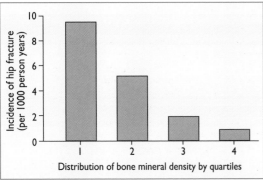

Association between bone density of femoral neck and risk of hip fracture. The quarter of patients with lowest bone density had 8·5 times higher risk of fracture than the quarter with highest bone density.

Preventing falls—Predisposing factors, such as postural hypotension or drowsiness due to drugs, should be eliminated. Patients should receive physiotherapy to improve their balance and righting reflexes. Hip protectors, designed to absorb the impact of a fall onto the hip, have been shown to reduce the incidence of hip fracture among residents of nursing homes. Patients should be provided with appropriate walking aids, and an environmental assessment should be made of their accommodation to eliminate hazards such as loose mats and cables.

Drug treatments should be monitored by measuring bone density since some patients fail to respond to certain drugs. There is little evidence that the rate of bone loss is accelerated once treatment is stopped.

Preventing osteoporosis

The aim in prevention should be to increase peak bone mass and to reduce subsequent rate of bone loss. Hormone replacement therapy is the most effective preventative measure against osteoporosis. Prophylactic treatment against bone loss should be targeted towards postmenopausal women whose bone mineral density at the lumbar spine or hip is more than one standard deviation below the mean for their age. Women with bone mineral density above the mean for young adults probably do not require hormone replacement therapy for prevention of osteoporosis. Women with intermediate bone densities may benefit from hormone replacement treatment if they lose bone at a faster rate than average. This may be determined from a repeat measurement of bone mineral density after two years. It may be possible in future to predict who will lose bone quickly by means of biochemical markers of bone turnover.

Further information

Further information about osteoporosis, including information for patients and details of patient support groups, is available from:

- The National Osteoporosis Society
  PO Box 10, Radstock, Bath BA3 3YB
  Telephone (01761) 471771, fax (01761) 471104
  Helpline (01761) 472721.

The scanning electron micrographs were prepared by Professor P Motta, Department of Anatomy, University "La Sapienza," Rome, and are reproduced with permission of the Science Photo Library. The photograph of kyphosis was prepared by John Radcliffe Hospital and is reproduced with permission of the Science Photo Library. The sources of the data presented in graphs are: B L Riggs and L J Melton, *N Engl J Med* 1986; **314**: 1676–86 for the incidence of osteoporotic fractures with age; and S R Cummings *et al*, *Lancet* 1993; **341**: 72–5 for the incidence of hip fracture by bone density. The data are reproduced with permission of the journals.

10 RHEUMATOID ARTHRITIS: CLINICAL FEATURES AND DIAGNOSIS

M Akil, R S Amos

Rheumatoid arthritis is the commonest disorder of connective tissues and is an important cause of disability, morbidity, and mortality. Life expectancy is reduced by four years in men and by 10 years in women, though this reduction is accounted for by a minority of patients with more severe disease. Nevertheless, patients with this condition may be offered life insurance only on the basis of loaded premiums.

Rheumatoid arthritis occurs worldwide with variable incidence and severity. In Western countries, it affects up to 1–3% of the population, although many are not severely affected and may not seek medical advice at all. Overall, there is a 3:1 female preponderance, but this excess is greater in young people and the age related incidence is approximately equal in elderly people.

The aetiology of rheumatoid arthritis remains unclear, but there is evidence of genetic predisposition to the disease. The presence of HLA-DR4 is significantly commoner among sufferers of rheumatoid arthritis who are white. Rheumatoid arthritis is associated with only certain subtypes of HLA-DR4 (HLA-Dw4 and HLA-Dw14); susceptibility is related to a shared epitope on the HLA molecule.

Factors associated with poorer prognosis in rheumatoid arthritis

- Insidious polyarticular onset
- Male patients
- Extra-articular manifestations
- Functional disability at one year after start of disease
- Substantially raised concentration of rheumatoid factors
- Presence of HLA-DR4
- Radiographic evidence of erosions within three years of start of disease

---

Rheumatoid arthritis in women

- Higher incidence of disease in women of child bearing age
- Disease tends to go into remission during pregnancy and to flare after giving birth
- Use of contraceptive pill or high gravidity adds some protection against later development of disease

---

Clinical features

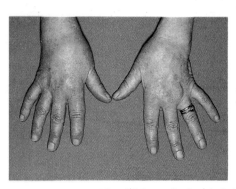 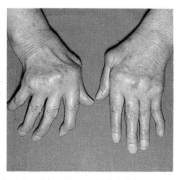

Effect of rheumatoid arthritis on the hand: (left) early changes and (right) later deformity.

Causes of impaired hand function in rheumatoid arthritis

- Active synovitis
- Joint deformity
- Rupture of tendon
- Carpal tunnel syndrome
- Mononeuritis
- Compression of nerve root at T1
- Compression of spinal cord

Joint damage

The start of the disease is usually insidious but can be episodic or acute. Rheumatoid arthritis usually presents as a polyarthritis affecting small joints or small and large joints. Early disease is characterised by pain and other cardinal signs of inflammation (heat, swelling, functional loss, and possible erythema over the joints) but not by damage and deformity. If the disease remains active and uncontrolled the inflammation will usually spread to additional joints and gradual irreversible tissue damage will occur, causing deformity and instability of joints. The most serious long term disability is associated with damage to the larger weight bearing joints.

Inflammation of other synovial structures is common, and a similar process may occur in tendon sheaths, progressing to serious dysfunction and rupture. The typical rheumatoid deformities—such as ulnar deviation of the fingers, z deformity of the thumb, and swan neck and boutonnière deformities—are mostly due to damage or displacement of tendons. Palpable thickening or nodularity of tendons is common.

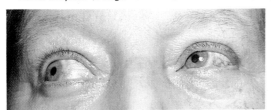

Magnetic resonance image of cervical spine showing spinal cord compression at C1 and C2.

Extra-articular manifestations of rheumatoid arthritis

- *Rheumatoid nodules*
- *Vasculitis*
- *Pulmonary*
  Pleural effusion
    Fibrosing alveolitis
    Nodules
- *Cardiac*
  Pericarditis
  Mitral valve disease
  Conduction defects
- *Skin*
  Palmar erythema
  Cutaneous vasculitis
  Pyoderma gangrenosum

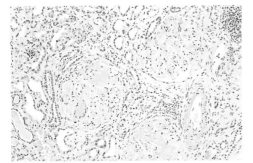

Renal amyloid (Congo red stain).

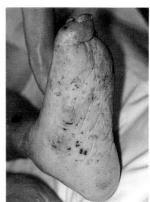

Scleritis associated with rheumatoid arthritis.

Complications of rheumatoid arthritis

- Joint failure causing physical disability
- Osteoporosis
- Depression
- Increased risk of infections
- Amyloidosis
- Complications of medical and surgical treatment

The spine—Although rheumatoid arthritis predominantly affects peripheral joints, discovertebral joints of the cervical spine are often affected. This may lead to atlantoaxial subluxation or, less commonly, subluxation at lower levels, with subsequent compression of the spinal cord. The earliest and most common symptom of cervical subluxation is pain radiating up into the occiput. Other symptoms include paraesthesia, sudden deterioration in hand function, sensory loss, abnormal gait, and urinary retention or incontinence.

Effusion of the knee may produce a popliteal (Baker's) cyst. This may rupture to cause diffuse pain and swelling in the calf that mimics deep vein thrombosis.

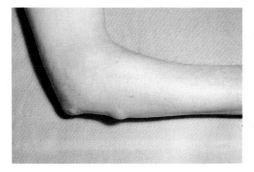

Rheumatoid nodule (above) and rheumatoid vasculitis (right).

Non-articular manifestations

Non-articular manifestations of rheumatoid arthritis are common. Rheumatoid nodules—which affect about a fifth of patients—may occur anywhere but are most common at sites of pressure, notably the extensor surfaces of the forearms and the posterior surface of the Achilles tendon.

A wide variety of other systems may be damaged by the rheumatoid process. Disease of small and sometimes larger blood vessels may be caused by deposition of immune complex in the vascular walls. This can lead to digital infarction, larger skin ulcers, and mononeuritis because of damage to the vasa nervorum.

Renal disease is rare but may occur as a result of amyloidosis, which presents as proteinuria or drug toxicity.

Eye complications

Sjögren's syndrome—The sicca complex results in dry gritty eyes with slight redness but normal vision. It is confirmed with the Schirmer test, which measures the wetting of a strip of sterilised filter paper when one end is placed under the eyelid. It is usually a late feature in women with seropositive rheumatoid arthritis.

Episcleritis is ocular irritation with nodules. Vision is normal.

Scleritis causes severe pain and occasionally reduces vision. There is diffuse or nodular redness, and the end stage of the condition is healing, with atrophy producing a bluish-grey sclera.

Felty's syndrome

This is a combination of seropositive rheumatoid arthritis (often with relatively inactive synovitis) with splenomegaly and neutropenia. It is associated with serious infections, vasculitis (leg ulcers, mononeuritis), anaemia, thrombocytopenia, and lymphadenopathy.

Neurological complications

These include entrapment of peripheral nerves (carpal tunnel, ulnar, lateral popliteal, tarsal, etc); mononeuritis multiplex; peripheral neuropathy—either associated with the disease or caused by drugs; compression of nerve roots; and compression of the cervical region of the spinal cord.

Investigations

Laboratory findings in rheumatoid arthritis

- Anaemia—normochromic or hypochromic, normocytic (if microcytic consider iron deficiency)
- Thrombocytosis
- Raised erythrocyte sedimentation rate
- Raised C reactive protein concentration
- Raised ferritin concentration as acute phase protein
- Low serum iron concentration
- Low total iron binding capacity
- Raised serum globulin concentrations
- Raised serum alkaline phosphatase activity
- Presence of rheumatoid factor

Other causes of positive test for rheumatoid factor

- Other connective tissue diseases
- Viral infections
- Leprosy
- Leishmaniasis
- Subacute bacterial endocarditis
- Tuberculosis
- Liver diseases
- Sarcoidosis
- Mixed essential cryoglobulinaemia

Causes of anaemia in rheumatoid arthritis

- Anaemia of chronic disease
- Iron deficiency—blood loss caused by non-steroidal anti-inflamatory drugs
- Suppression of bone marrow function—caused by sulphasalazine, penicillamine, gold, and cytotoxic drugs
- Folate deficiency—caused by sulphasalazine, methotrexate
- Vitamin B-12 deficiency—caused by associated pernicious anaemia
- Haemolysis—caused by sulphasalazine and dapsone
- Felty's syndrome

Radiograph of hands showing rheumatoid erosions.

Immune abnormalities

Rheumatoid factors are anti-immunoglobulins, and anti-IgG IgM is the immunological hallmark of rheumatoid arthritis. It is detected with the Rose-Waaler assay, but it is neither universally present in, nor specific for, rheumatoid arthritis: it is found in the sera of 80% of patients with rheumatoid arthritis, but the remainder are persistently seronegative despite otherwise typical disease. These patients may, however, be found to carry rheumatoid factors of other isotypes. The extra-articular features of rheumatoid arthritis are much commoner in patients with high concentrations of rheumatoid factor, but it is a poor guide to the severity of joint disease and to the success or otherwise of treatment.

Antinuclear antibodies may be present in some patients. The test for antinuclear antibody is widely used to screen for systemic lupus erythematosus, but it should be remembered that some patients with lupus will have positive tests for rheumatoid factor while some patients with rheumatoid arthritis will have positive tests for antinuclear antibody. Thus neither test is a universal diagnostic tool.

Indicators of acute phase response

A raised eryhrocyte sedimentation rate (or plasma viscosity) and the presence of acute phase proteins such as C reactive protein are commonly found in patients with rheumatoid arthritis, especially when the disease is active. They reflect the severity of acute inflammation and thus may be a reasonable guide to the success of drug treatment, though they are not specific to rheumatoid arthritis. The disease is likely to progress if a raised erythrocyte sedimentation rate (or presence of C reactive protein) persists, but progression can still occur if they do not persist.

Liver function

Tests for liver function may give abnormal results in patients with rheumatoid arthritis. Serum concentrations of transaminases and alkaline phosphatase may be moderately elevated when the disease is active.

Radiography

Radiographs of the hands often are normal at presentation or may show swelling of soft tissue, loss of joint space, or periarticular osteoporosis. Erosions typical of rheumatoid arthritis develop within three years of the start of the disease in over 90% of patients who ultimately develop the erosions.

Unusual presentations

Unusual patterns of start of rheumatoid arthritis
• Palindromic   • Polymyalgic • Monoarthritic   • Oligoarthritic • Asymmetrical

Differential diagnosis of rheumatoid arthritis
Psoriatic arthritis—always seronegative Primary nodal osteoarthritis Other connective tissue diseases Calcium pyrophosphate deposition disease

Symmetrical small joint polyarthritis, with or without large joints also being affected, is the commonest presentation. In elderly patients the start of rheumatoid arthritis may be indistinguishable from polymyalgia rheumatica. Occasionally, rheumatoid arthritis may present as a monoarthritis. Other conditions (such as infection, crystal arthritis, other inflammatory arthritis, etc) must be excluded before a diagnosis of rheumatoid arthritis is made.

Palindromic rheumatism is characterised by recurrent episodes of mostly oligoarticular arthritis that leave no residual clinical or radiological changes. Up to half of patients with this condition later develop typical rheumatoid arthritis, often accompanied by conversion to seropositivity for rheumatoid factor.

11 RHEUMATOID ARTHRITIS: TREATMENT

M Akil, R S Amos

Except for the mildest cases, rheumatoid arthritis cannot be adequately managed by one specialist in isolation from others. Most people with rheumatoid arthritis cope better if they understand their condition and have realistic expectations of the benefits and disadvantages of treatment. Therefore, education of patients is an important aspect of treatment. Specialist rheumatology nurses have become well established in many rheumatology departments; their role includes monitoring drugs used to treat rheumatoid arthritis and differentiating minor or unrelated symptoms from those that require action.

Physical therapy

In a physiotherapy department local measures such as heat, cold, and electrotherapy may be used to reduce pain and generally form part of a rehabilitation programme of exercises designed to improve muscle strength and encourage mobility in affected joints. The aims of occupational therapy are to educate patients; to protect joints; to analyse function and to improve it by means of exercise and use of aids and appliances; and to provide splints when necessary.

Few of the individual techniques used in physiotherapy and occupational therapy have been subjected to controlled trials, but there is no doubt that therapists who are skilled in handling atrophied, inflamed, and stiff tissues and are familiar with the problems faced by patients with arthritis greatly help in treatment and rehabilitation.

Surgery

The aims of surgery are to relieve pain and to restore function. Indications for urgent treatment are septic arthritis, ruptured tendons, and compression of nerves and spinal cord.

Although synovectomy may slow down damage for a relatively short period, it does not alter the final outcome. This procedure is becoming less popular among surgeons who specialise in treating arthritis. When surgery is being considered the patient must be part of the decision making process, as must the patient's rheumatologist as well as the surgeon, and should have a realistic understanding of the procedure. The timing of surgery is crucial: for example, forefoot arthroplasty, if indicated, should usually precede knee or hip arthroplasty to minimise the risk of infection.

Drugs for relief of symptoms

Side effects of non-steroidal anti-inflammatory drugs

- *Gastrointestinal tract*
Dyspepsia and gastritis
Gastric or duodenal ulceration
Diarrhoea
Hepatitis
- *Central nervous system*
Headache and dizziness
Tinnitus
Confusion
Aseptic meningitis
- *Cardiovascular system*
Oedema
Hypertension
Heart failure
- *Respiratory system*
Asthma
Pneumonitis
- *Blood*
Neutropenia
Thrombocytopenia
Aplastic anaemia
Haemolytic anaemia
- *Kidney*
Precipitation of acute renal failure
Haematuria
Nephrotic syndrome
Papillary necrosis
Interstitial nephritis
- *Hypersensitivity reactions*

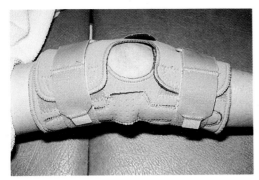

Braces help to reduce instability of damaged joints.

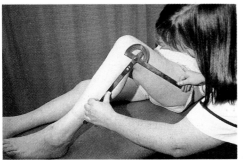

Assessment and measurement of range of movement of joint.

Non-steroidal anti-inflammatory drugs

These drugs provide symptomatic relief but do not modify the course of the disease. For the mildest cases they may be used alone, but they are usually used in combination with disease modifying drugs. The response of individual patients varies, and several drugs may be tried in succession to find a suitable one. A single large dose at night, especially if the drug is in a slow release form, often helps to relieve early morning stiffness.

Gastrointestinal toxicity is the commonest side effect. Inflammation, erosion, and ulceration occur in the oesophagus, stomach, duodenum, and small bowel. These are often chronic and asymptomatic, presenting with anaemia or occasionally with acute upper gastrointestinal bleeding. H_2 blockers reduce the risk of duodenal ulceration but have little protective effect against gastric ulcers. Misoprostol, a synthetic analogue of prostaglandin E1, protects against gastric and duodenal ulcers, but its use is limited by the high incidence of diarrhoea and abdominal pain. It should not be used in women who are or may become pregnant. Proton pump inhibitors are used for gastro-oesophageal reflux, which can be exacerbated by non-steroidal anti-inflammatory drugs. Routine prophylaxis against peptic ulcer disease is controversial, but it is required for patients with a previous history of ulceration.

Non-steroidal anti-inflammatory drugs should be used with caution in patients with renal failure, cardiac failure, or uncontrolled hypertension to avoid decompensation due to renal prostanoid blockade. Interstitial nephritis may present idiosyncratically. Concomitant administration of non-steroidal anti-inflammatory drugs with anticoagulants is best avoided if possible.

Administration of non-steroidal anti-inflammatory drugs in the later stages of pregnancy delays the onset and increases the duration of labour. It may lead to the closure of ductus arteriosus in utero and possibly persistent pulmonary hypertension of the newborn. The drugs are safe for use by lactating mothers except for aspirin, which may increase the risk of Reye's syndrome in children.

Simple analgesia

Paracetamol, dextropropoxyphene, and codeine are used for simple pain relief. The choice is not critical but depends on patients' preferences. Stronger, narcotic analgesics should be avoided.

Corticosteroids

Intra-articular corticosteroids can help to settle a flare. Long acting (depot) drugs such as triamcinolone or methylprednisolone are usually used for injection of large joints, but hydrocortisone or prednisolone is preferable for superficial joints or flexor tendon sheaths because of the lower incidence of subcutaneous and skin atrophy.

Bolus intravenous or intramuscular corticosteroids can be used as an adjunct to the slower acting second line drugs. This procedure has not become popular, but it may be suitable for managing some of the systemic complications of rheumatoid arthritis. The potential hazards include avascular bone necrosis, spread of systemic sepsis, and cardiac arrhythmias.

Daily oral corticosteroids—Such regular use of corticosteroids for rheumatoid synovitis is controversial. There is speculation about whether corticosteroids may modify the disease process and, if so, whether this can be achieved in small doses. Prednisolone should be used as an early treatment for rheumatoid arthritis only in cases of severe disability due to persistent disease activity and as an adjunct to treatment with second line drugs. Continual corticosteroid treatment exacerbates the local and systemic osteopenia that accompanies active and chronic rheumatoid arthritis, and no dose avoids risk.

Drugs that suppress the disease process

These drugs play a key role in the treatment of rheumatoid arthritis, and recent recommendations have focused on their early and continued use. This is because of the serious long term outcome of rheumatoid arthritis and therefore the need to intervene early with the most effective drugs. All these drugs are potentially toxic, and regular monitoring for toxicity is necessary. There is considerable variation in the monitoring schedules followed by different rheumatologists, and those given below reflect the authors' experience and practice.

Sulphasalazine

This is a popular first choice drug. Benefit develops progressively after about six weeks, so a non-steroidal anti-inflammatory drug should be continued. About 60% of patients given the drug continue taking it after three years, while it is withdrawn in 15% because of toxicity.

The irritating, though rarely serious, side effects include nausea, headache, and abdominal discomfort, and the incidence of such side effects is probably reduced by the use of enteric coated tablets. A skin rash is occasionally a problem, and the drug should not be used for patients who are allergic to sulphonamides.

Bone marrow toxicity and hepatitis are among the more serious side effects. These are more common in the first six months of treatment. Patients' blood count and liver function should be checked before starting treatment, at monthly intervals for the first three months, and then once every three to six months. Other side effects include reversible oligospermia and, since sulphasalazine is excreted in most body fluids, yellow discoloration of urine and soft contact lenses.

Antimalarial drugs

These are less effective but safer than some other disease modifying drugs. Retinopathy is the main serious side effect and is commoner with chloroquine than hydroxychloroquine. Ophthalmic monitoring is advisable.

Penicillamine

This has a wide variety of potential side effects. A metallic taste and nausea are common early problems but resolve with continued use. Skin rashes, bone marrow toxicity, and proteinuria are more serious. Monitoring of blood and urine should initially be monthly; the interval is often increased thereafter, but toxicity may develop at any time.

Gold

Injectable gold (sodium aurothiomalate) can cause remission of rheumatoid arthritis, but the chances of tolerating long term treatment are modest. The commonest adverse reactions are skin rashes, but not all such rashes require a permanent end of treatment. Proteinuria can be the precursor to serious renal problems; if persistent, it should be investigated and gold treatment withheld. Blood dyscrasia is potentially lethal; the data sheet recommends that a blood count be obtained before each injection, but this is not always practical and many rheumatologists consider regular blood monitoring to be sufficient.

Auranofin is an oral preparation of gold. Diarrhoea is more common but is not a major problem, although it often leads to discontinuation of the drug. It is less effective than injectable gold, and the two drugs should not be regarded as interchangeable. Regular monitoring of blood and urine is necessary.

Azathioprine

This is used for synovitis and systemic complications of rheumatoid arthritis. The main initial limiting factor is nausea. Regular blood monitoring is necessary for early detection of bone marrow toxicity or derangement of liver function. Prolonged treatment may be associated with an increased risk of lymphoma. The usual dose is 2·5 mg/kg daily.

Treatment schedule for sulphasalazine

- Starting dose of 0·5 g or 1·0 g daily
- Increased over 3–4 weeks *to*
- Maintenance dose of 2·0 g daily
- After 3 months dose may be increased further to 2·5–3·0 g daily if required (and tolerated)

Desensitisation of patients who are allergic to sulphasalazine is possible by use of a series of very low doses of increasing strength (this is available in a special pack)

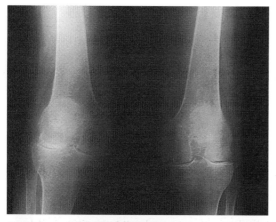

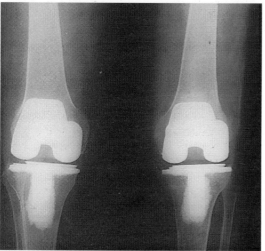

Radiographs showing knee joints with advanced arthritis (top) and their total replacement with prosthetic joints (bottom).

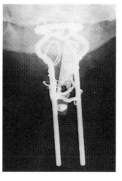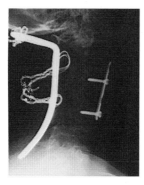

Frontal and side views of cervical spine fusion to treat subluxation.

Methotrexate

This has been used predominantly in North America and, more recently, in Europe in small once weekly oral or injectable doses. This regimen has helped many patients with rheumatoid arthritis, and in some centres methotrexate is the disease modifying drug of choice.

The most common side effect is nausea, which is not usually severe and may settle. More serious side effects include bone marrow toxicity and alveolitis. The risk of hepatic fibrosis and possibly cirrhosis seems to be extremely low in patients given intermittent low doses, though it should be used with reluctance in people who have more than a modest intake of alcohol. The need for regular liver biopsies is debatable, but they are hard to justify in patients with low risk.

How much immunosuppressant effect methotrexate actually has in intermittent low doses is debatable. There may be an increased risk of certain viral infections and possibly a slightly higher risk of some bacterial infections. If antibiotics are needed it seems important to avoid co-trimoxazole and probably trimethoprim. Certainly, the former can precipitate a blood dyscrasia, probably because of folic acid deficiency in patients taking methotrexate. A case could be made out for giving all such patients folic acid supplements. Certainly, red cell folate or at least mean corpuscular volume should be regularly monitored.

Cyclophosphamide

This has been used to treat severe rheumatoid synovitis resistant to other treatments and to treat systemic vasculitis. It carries the risk of all the side effects of immunosuppressive drugs and very careful monitoring is mandatory. Patients must understand the risk involved.

New and experimental treatments

Cyclosporin is expensive and potentially toxic, with a 40% risk of renal impairment and hypertension. It is best reserved for patients resistant to other drugs. Treatments to target specific immune mediated changes in rheumatoid arthritis are currently being investigated. The value of these treatments has not yet been established, but initial results are promising.

> ### Experimental treatments targeting specific immune mediated changes in rheumatoid arthritis
>
> * Cytokine inhibitors—such as recombinant human interleukin I receptor antagonist
> * Recombinant soluble tumour necrosis factor receptor
> * Antibodies to tumour necrosis factor α
> * Antibodies to CD4 cells

Complementary medicine

Since there is no cure for rheumatoid arthritis with conventional treatment, many patients turn to complementary medicine. Some of the treatments available are getting closer to the practice of orthodox medicine. Patients may take supplements to their diet or may turn to homoeopathy or, more recently, reflexology or iridology.

Diet

For centuries sufferers from rheumatic disease have been advised to alter their diet in the hope of improving their condition. There is no evidence that this changes the natural course of the disease, but some symptomatic relief might be obtained. Whether the basis of diet therapy lies in supplements of trace elements or antioxidants or in avoiding "toxic" or "allergenic" constituents remains to be determined. However, there is evidence that starvation produces short term improvement in the activity of rheumatoid arthritis, and this raises the possibility that dietary manipulation may have something to offer.

Dietary therapy involves the avoidance of foods thought to worsen synovitis, particularly dairy products, cereals, and eggs. An elimination diet consists of "non-allergenic" foods such as rice, carrots, and fish followed by graded reintroduction of other foods. Whichever way the diet is pursued, it is important that suspected foodstuffs are tested by repeated reintroduction. Extreme dietary exclusions may induce deficiency disorders.

Food supplements—A wide variety of supplements have been tried by patients suffering from rheumatoid arthritis, some of which may have anti-inflammatory properties. The benefits for rheumatoid arthritis that are claimed have yet to be proved.

> ### Food supplements claimed to help people with rheumatoid arthritis
>
> * Selenium supplements
> * Extracts from New Zealand green lipped mussel
> * Fish oil
> * Evening primrose oil

---

12 SPONDYLOARTHROPATHIES

Andrew Keat

Principal clinical features associated with spondyloarthropathies

Musculoskeletal
- Peripheral arthritis
- Enthesopathy
- Sacroiliitis
- Spondylitis

Systemic
- Psoriasis
- Inflammatory bowel disease
- Conjunctivitis and iritis
- Genitourinary inflammation
- Carditis

The spondyloarthropathies are a cluster of overlapping forms of inflammatory arthritis that are distinct from rheumatoid arthritis and characteristically affect the spine and entheses (insertions of tendons and ligaments). The syndromes include ankylosing spondylitis, reactive arthritis and Reiter's syndrome, psoriatic arthritis, and enteropathic arthritis. The arthropathy of Whipple's disease and Behçet's syndrome may also be included, although these are more controversial. Less clearly defined overlap categories also exist.

The spondyloarthropathies are distinguished by familial clusters of cases and a strong association with the class I histocompatibility molecules HLA-B27 and, to a lesser extent, HLA-CW6. However, tissue typing for HLA-B27 is not usually helpful and is not a reliable guide to prognosis. Unlike most patients with rheumatoid arthritis, patients with spondyloarthropathies are seronegative for anti-immunoglobulins (rheumatoid factors).

Spondyloarthropathies may present at any age, though young adults are primarily affected. In contrast with rheumatoid disease, both sexes are affected more or less equally, though with a slight male predominance. Spinal symptoms may also be more prominent in males.

Estimated prevalence of spondyloarthropathies and related conditions in United Kingdom

Disease	No of cases (per 100 000)	Male:female ratio
Ankylosing spondylitis	150	2·5
Psoriasis	2000	1·0
Psoriatic arthritis	20–100	1·3
Reactive arthritis and Reiter's syndrome	16	3·0
Ulcerative colitis	50–100	0·8
Crohn's disease	30–75	1·0
Enteropathic arthritis	1–20% of inflammatory bowel disease	*

* Peripheral arthritis occurs more often in women, while sacroiliitis and spondylitis occur more often in men.

Lesions

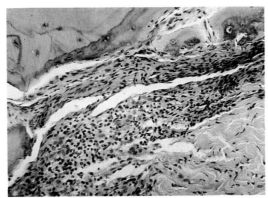

Histological section through enthesis showing cellular infiltrate between collagen bundles of fascia and periosteum: site of attachment is replaced by granulation tissue infiltrated by lymphocytes, plasma cells, and polymorphonuclear leucocytes. Deep to the superficial lesion there is also infiltration of the marrow space with inflammatory cells and oedema.

Entheses

The characteristic lesions of entheses — such as of the plantar fascia and Achilles tendon insertion — may appear as radiographic erosions. Repair by reactive bone leads to a new, more superficial enthesis, forming a bony spur. This is remodelled with cancellous bone, which eventually leads to ankylosis. Widespread diffuse lesions in the spine or pelvis may produce insidious stiffness and generalised discomfort.

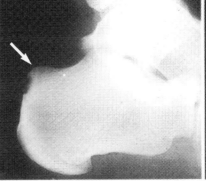
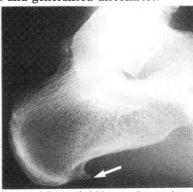

Radiographs of enthesis lesions: (left) enthesopathies at Achilles tendon and plantar fascia attachments to calcaneum, with local osteopenia appearing as erosions; (right) plantar calcaneal spur.

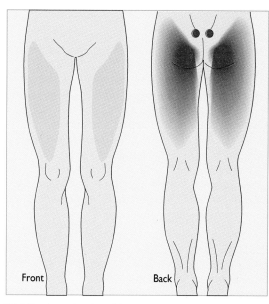

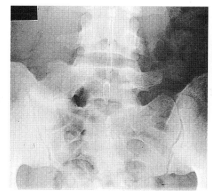 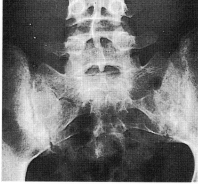

Radiographs showing appearance of normal sacroiliac joints (left) and of sacroiliitis (right).

Front   Back

Distribution of pain with sacroiliitis.

Sacroiliitis and spondylitis

Sacroiliitis most commonly presents as bilateral or unilateral discomfort in the buttocks, usually worse after inactivity but sometimes aggravated by weight bearing. Diagnosis may be missed unless other clinical features are present. It is important to distinguish sacroiliitis from referred lumbosacral pain.

Techniques for imaging sacroiliac joints

	Benefits	Shortcomings
Radiography*	Quick and cheap	Changes occur late
Radionuclide imaging	May indicate early changes	Controversial; of uncertain value in the adolescent skeleton
Computed tomography	Clear imaging of early changes May clarify diagnosis when radiographs equivocal	Changes occur late
Magnetic resonance imaging	Best technique for early diagnosis	Price and availability

* Oblique view — prone view with beam angled 15° down.

Sacroiliitis principally affects the lower anterior synovial portion of the joint. Early changes include juxta-articular osteoporosis associated with osteitis and bony overgrowth over the anterior and posterior aspect of the joint — capsular enthesopathy. This may be reflected on radiographs by widening of the sacroiliac joint with marginal sclerosis. Later, juxta-articular sclerosis and subsequent obliteration of the joint occur. Computed tomography may show erosive changes not clearly visible on radiographs, and magnetic resonance imaging may show early juxta-articular osteitis.

Peripheral synovitis

Peripheral synovitis is characterised by its clinical distribution and by relatively good prognosis compared with rheumatoid disease. When small joints are affected generally only one or a few joints in the same extremity are affected. Synovitis of finger joints is associated with psoriasis, although only 10% of patients have typical involvement of distal interphalangeal joints with nail pitting. Psoriasis and joint damage may be especially severe in patients infected with HIV. Transient disease is often non-erosive, but persistent synovitis may result in articular erosions, particularly at small joints. Synovitis is indistinguishable histologically and immunohistochemically from typical rheumatoid disease.

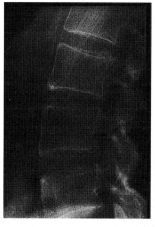 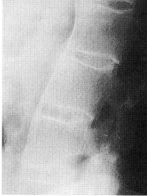

Radiographs showing lumbar vertebral squaring in early spondylitis (left) and spinal fusion in late spondylitis (right).

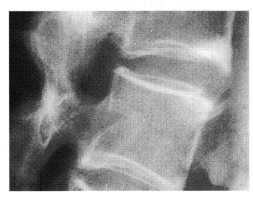

Radiograph showing marginal syndesmophyte formation in established spondylitis. Spondylitis may affect all parts of the spine except for the atlantoaxial joint, where mobility is maintained.

Eye lesions

Synchronous conjunctivitis occurs in a third of patients with reactive arthritis, and acute anterior uveitis occurs in 4–5% of patients with spondyloarthropathies at some time. The two conditions are indistinguishable clinically, and slit lamp examination is necessary. Red, sore, or gritty eyes or blurring of vision need urgent ophthalmological examination. Acute anterior uveitis does not usually occur in synchrony with flares of arthritis.

Spondyloarthropathies

Gut lesions

Various lesions, which may be subclinical, have been described in association with spondyloarthropathies. Indeed, subtle inflammatory changes in both small and large bowel are present in a substantial proportion of patients with established spondyloarthropathy syndromes.

Genitourinary lesions

Sexually transmitted infection of the lower genital tract is well recognised in the initiation of reactive arthritis. Urethritis and cervicitis may also accompany arthritis after acute bacterial diarrhoea, and prostatitis and salpingitis have been linked with spondylitis. Psoriasiform lesions over the external genitalia (circinate balanitis and circinate vulvitis) do not relate directly to the presence of genitourinary infection.

Syndromes

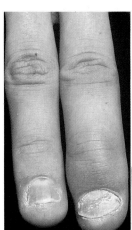

Psoriatic arthritis: typical swelling of distal interphalangeal joint with nail dystrophy.

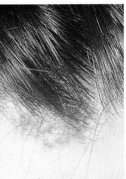

Easily missed psoriatic lesions in scalp (left) and natal cleft (right).

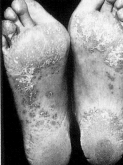
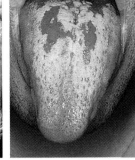

Psoriatic lesions: on feet, identical to keratoderma blennorrhagica (left); on tongue (right).

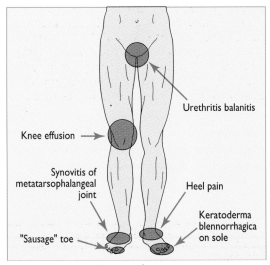

Characteristic distribution of clinical lesions in reactive arthritis.

Urethritis balanitis

Knee effusion

Synovitis of metatarsophalangeal joint

Heel pain

Keratoderma blennorrhagica on sole

"Sausage" toe

Ankylosing spondylitis

The New York criteria (1966) for the diagnosis of ankylosing spondylitis require a combination of clinical and radiographic features, but the diagnosis should be suspected on the basis of inactivity, spinal stiffness, and pain, with or without additional features.

Psoriatic arthritis

This is an inflammatory arthritis — usually with negative tests for IgM rheumatoid factor — with coincidental psoriasis. Plaque, guttate, or pustular psoriasis — with or without nail involvement — may precede or follow the start of arthritis, which is a distinct entity. Five different patterns of arthritis are recognised: monoarthritis and oligoarthritis, polyarthritis, inflammation of distal interphalangeal joints and nail dystrophy, arthritis mutilans, and spondylitis. As well as typical oligoarticular peripheral arthritis, the upper limbs are commonly affected, with both arthritis and dactylitis and in some patients a rheumatoid arthritis-like polyarthritis (rheumatoid factor negative).

A search for psoriasis should include the scalp, natal cleft, and feet. Mucosal psoriatic lesions may affect the genitalia and tongue. Lesions may be especially severe and widespread in patients infected with HIV.

Enteropathic arthritis

Enteropathic arthritis is peripheral or axial arthritis occurring in association with ulcerative colitis or Crohn's disease. Inflammatory bowel lesions are associated with the development of both spondylitis and peripheral arthritis, even in the absence of HLA-B27.

Reactive arthritis and Reiter's syndrome

These two terms refer to different aspects of the same condition, so that debate over which term to use is not particularly helpful.

Reiter's syndrome was originally defined as the triad of arthritis, conjunctivitis, and inflammation of the genital tract, but it has been defined more recently by the American Rheumatism Association as an episode of peripheral arthritis of more than one month's duration occurring in association with urethritis or cervicitis, or both.

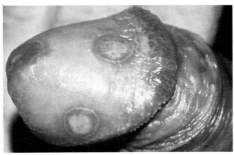

Circinate balanitis: mucosal psoriasis typical of reactive arthritis.

Reactive arthritis refers to non-septic arthritis strongly linked to a recognised episode of infection. Arthritis may be described as reactive if it is associated with bacterial infection at a distant site but viable micro-micro-organisms are not present in the affected joint. This term is therefore equally applicable to rheumatic fever, arthritis after meningococcaemia, and Reiter's syndrome after dysentery.

Unfortunately it is still difficult to find suitable terms to adequately describe disease suffered by many individual patients. The terms sexually acquired reactive arthritis (SARA) and enteric reactive arthritis (ERA) have been introduced to allow accurate categorisation of conditions associated with infections at specific sites. Such descriptions are likely to be supplanted as understanding of pathogenesis improves.

Infection

Micro-organisms linked with reactive arthritis

Genitourinary	Gastrointestinal	Other
Chlamydia trachomatis	Clostridium difficile	Chlamydia pneumoniae
Ureaplasma urealyticum	Entamoeba histolytica	Streptococcus pyogenes
Neisseria gonorrhoeae	Giardia lamblia	Borrelia burgdorferi
	Shigella spp	Blastocystis hominis
	Escherichia coli (enterotoxicogenic strains)	
	Yersinia spp	
	Campylobacter jejuni	
	Salmonella spp	

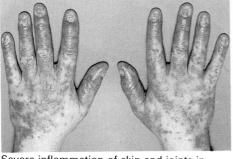

Severe inflammation of skin and joints in patient with psoriatic arthritis and AIDS.

Several gut and genitourinary pathogens are known to trigger reactive arthritis, and others have been more tenuously linked. Recent reports have suggested that respiratory tract infections by streptococci and *Chlamydia pneumoniae* may be associated with the development of oligoarticular arthritis.

Some patients with acute reactive arthritis also develop sacroiliitis or spondylitis, either synchronously or subsequently, but in most patients with spondyloarthritis there is no clear evidence of infection. Evidence of cross reactivity between a klebsiella microbial protein and parts of the B27 molecule has been found, but there is no conclusive evidence of a role for this micro-organism in the aetiology of spondylitis.

HIV infection

Arthritis, including typical reactive arthritis, certainly occurs in patients infected with HIV or with AIDS, and both joint lesions and psoriasis may be exceptionally severe. There is, however, no clear evidence that HIV infection itself constitutes a risk factor for spondyloarthropathies. In contrast septic bone and joint lesions do occur more commonly in patients with AIDS, as their CD4 cell count falls. It is, therefore, crucial to consider the possibility of septic arthritis by both common and opportunistic infective agents in these patients.

Management

Treatment for spondyloarthropathies

Treatment	Indication	Caution
Physiotherapy	Spinal mobilisation, hydrotherapy in spondylitis, maintaining local muscle power (such as quadriceps)	Manipulation may be dangerous
Local steroid injection	To single inflamed joints, entheses, and bursae	Weight bearing enthesis Not more than three injections a year
Non-steroidal anti-inflammatory drugs	Spinal stiffness, pain, persistent synovitis or enthesopathy	Elderly patients, peptic ulcer, inflammatory bowel disease
Oral or systemic corticosteroid	Short courses for intolerable symptoms, uveitis	May precipitate heart failure and progressive osteoporosis
Sulphasalazine	Persistent aggressive disease	As for rheumatoid arthritis
Methotrexate	Persistent aggressive peripheral joint disease, possibly of value in axial disease	As for rheumatoid arthritis
Antibiotics	Acute infection of genital tract, persistent sexually associated reactive arthritis	Microbiological basis for treatment should be established

The objectives of treatment are relief of symptoms and maintenance of function. Anti-inflammatory drugs should be used to reduce pain and stiffness in order to permit proper mobilisation of joints. Physiotherapy, with daily exercises, is obligatory for patients with ankylosing spondylitis in order to prevent deformity of the spine, especially the neck.

The pictures showing histological appearance of an enthesis, site of pain in sacroiliitis, and radiographic appearance of early spondylitis are reproduced with permission of Gower Medical Publishing.

13 ARTHRITIS IN CHILDREN

T R Southwood

Rheumatic symptoms, such as limping or limb pain, are common in children, yet childhood arthritis and other rheumatic diseases are rare. Diagnosis and treatment of these conditions therefore require a high level of clinical awareness and careful assessment. Laboratory investigations are rarely pathognomonic and are used instead to help differential diagnosis, to detect complications, and to monitor disease activity. Drug treatment depends on a sound knowledge of the variable nature and prognosis of the conditions and a clear understanding of the pharmacology, risks, and benefits of anti-inflammatory and antirheumatic drugs in children.

Persistent swelling of joints characterises a heterogeneous group of diseases termed juvenile chronic arthritis, formerly known as Still's disease. This group of diseases is, for the most part, genetically and clinically distinct from rheumatoid arthritis in adults. About one child in every 1000 has juvenile chronic arthritis, amounting to over 12 000 affected children in Britain. Each year one new case would be expected in every 10 000 children.

Children with arthritis may not complain of pain, but most do experience some discomfort

The diagnosis of juvenile chronic arthritis is often difficult initially because swelling of joints may be subtle or absent and complaints of pain may be difficult to elicit from children. Children may present with limping, upper limb dysfunction, torticollis, or non-specific constitutional symptoms such as lethargy, fever, poor appetite, or irritability. Occasionally, features not associated with the musculoskeletal system may predominate: rash, pericarditis, serositis, or organomegaly. Prompt diagnosis and an early start of appropriate treatment are important; the longer the delay, the greater the risk of joint contractures, muscle wasting, and abnormal growth.

Common mistakes in diagnosis of juvenile chronic arthritis are:

Diagnosis in absence of persistent, objective joint swelling
Failure to exclude differential diagnoses

Classification of juvenile chronic arthritis

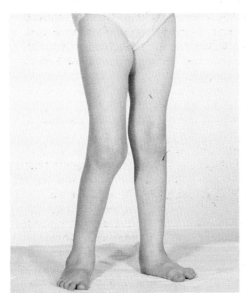

Juvenile chronic arthritis of pauciarticular onset of right knee in 3 year old girl.

The basis of the classification of juvenile chronic arthritis is the number of joints affected during the first six months of the disease and the presence of extra-articular clinical features. There are three main clinical patterns: pauciarticular onset affects up to four joints, polyarticular onset affects five or more joints, and systemic onset has prominent extra-articular features such as fever and rash.

Juvenile chronic arthritis of pauciarticular onset

This is the most common subtype of juvenile chronic arthritis, accounting for over half of cases, and usually affects young (preschool) girls. It is commonly associated with antinuclear antibodies. A fifth of patients develop the clinically silent but potentially blinding complication of chronic anterior uveitis. The articular prognosis for patients is good: in most cases the arthritis is not severe and only persists for a few years, although a third of patients will eventually develop polyarthritis that is difficult to control.

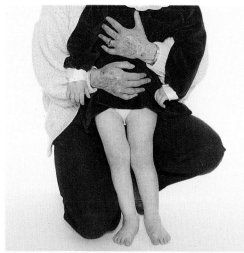

Juvenile chronic arthritis of pauciarticular onset of knee (and dactylitis of a finger) in child whose mother has psoriasis on dorsal surface of her hands.

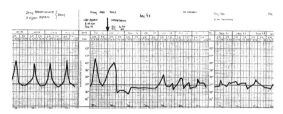

Temperature chart showing characteristic quotidian fever caused by juvenile chronic arthritis of systemic onset. The fever was uncontrolled by prednisolone 20 mg/day and high dose aspirin, but it settled after substitution with indomethacin 20 mg/kg/day.

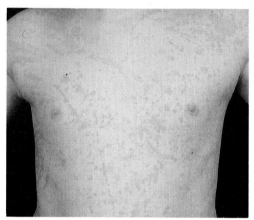

Typical erythematous evanescent rash of juvenile chronic arthritis of systemic onset. Often it is obvious only at the height of fever and is sometimes confined to the axillary region and lateral chest wall.

Two other groups of patients may also present with pauciarticular disease; those with juvenile psoriatic arthritis and those who are predisposed to ankylosing spondylitis. Both of these groups may be difficult to diagnose at the start of disease, as arthritis may predate by many years the characteristic clinical features of psoriasis or of sacroiliitis or spondyloarthritis. Clues to the diagnosis of juvenile psoriatic arthritis without a typical psoriatic rash are a family history of psoriasis, pitting of nails, and an asymmetrical arthritic pattern affecting both small joints (such as those of the finger) and large joints. Juvenile psoriatic arthritis seems to have a poorer prognosis than juvenile chronic arthritis of pauciarticular onset without psoriasis.

Children who are predisposed to ankylosing spondylitis are usually boys who develop a predominantly lower limb arthritis during late childhood or adolescence. An important clinical feature of such children is enthesitis—inflammation and tenderness at the site of insertion of tendons, ligaments, or fascia into bone. The most common clinically detectable sites of enthesitis are around the foot: the insertions of the plantar fascia into the calcaneum, the base of the fifth metatarsal and the metatarsal heads, and the insertion of the Achilles tendon into the calcaneum posteriorly. There is often a family history of "bad backs," inflammatory bowel disease, or acute uveitis. Although radiological evidence of sacroiliitis is rarely present at the start of this disease in children, over half will eventually develop ankylosing spondylitis.

Juvenile chronic arthritis of polyarticular onset

This arthritis, which is predominantly symmetrical and affects upper and lower limbs, is found in 30–40% of children with juvenile chronic arthritis. Most patients are girls who develop arthritis during their preschool years. However, the disease can also start in late childhood or adolescence, and such cases, which account for less than 10% of cases of juvenile chronic arthritis, are the only ones associated with persistent serological evidence of rheumatoid factor. This probably represents the juvenile manifestation of the adult type of rheumatoid arthritis. Both groups of patients with arthritis of polyarticular onset have a poorer articular prognosis than those with disease of pauciarticular onset; 30–50% develop bony erosions and active arthritis that persists into adulthood.

Juvenile chronic arthritis of systemic onset

This is the rarest form of juvenile chronic arthritis. Most patients develop the disease in early childhood, but patients of any age may be affected, including adults. It is often difficult to diagnose because the earliest features may be extra-articular. These include a characteristic fever; an evanescent, macular, erythematous rash; and evidence of serositis, organomegaly, or lymphadenopathy. The number of arthritic joints varies: about a third of patients develop severe polyarthritis that is resistant to treatment, and the articular outlook for these patients is poor. The life threatening complications of pericarditis and amyloidosis are associated with this disease.

Laboratory investigations

Key investigations for differential diagnosis of juvenile chronic arthritis

- Synovial fluid aspiration for microscopy and culture if sepsis is suspected
- Full blood count (and bone marrow aspiration if neoplasia is suspected)
- Measurement of acute phase proteins
- Plain radiographs of affected joint

No investigation is pathognomonic of juvenile chronic arthritis, but several are useful for differential diagnosis. Measures of the acute phase response (erythrocyte sedimentation rate, C reactive protein, and serum viscosity) are raised in about 70% of patients with juvenile chronic arthritis at diagnosis and are useful for monitoring disease activity. Antinuclear antibodies are found in about half of patients with juvenile chronic arthritis of pauciarticular onset, and their presence correlates with the risk of chronic anterior uveitis. Antinuclear antibodies are not, however, specific for this disease; they are also found in 20% of patients with polyarticular disease, 5% of those with systemic disease, patients with many other connective tissue diseases, and 5% of apparently normal children.

Arthritis in children

Tests for rheumatoid factor, synovial biopsy, and plain radiographs are unsuitable for use in screening. Rheumatoid factor is neither specific nor sensitive for chronic arthritis in children—it is absent in over 90% of patients with the disease—and is present in many patients with infectious and other inflammatory diseases. Synovial biopsy is useful to exclude diseases such as foreign body synovitis or tuberculous arthritis, but with juvenile chronic arthritis biopsy is usually non-specific and reveals only chronic inflammatory changes. Radiographic features of local bone pathology are useful for differential diagnosis of a swollen joint. Narrowing of joint spaces and bony erosions—two features of severe juvenile chronic arthritis—usually occur too late in the course of the disease to help in diagnosis.

Treatment

One of the most important factors in successful treatment of juvenile chronic arthritis is the expertise of nurses, physiotherapists, and occupational therapists in paediatric rheumatology

Complications of juvenile chronic arthritis

Pain and constitutional features
- Including lethargy, anorexia, and irritability

Joint contractures
- Pain caused by raised intra-articular pressure and muscle spasm may be contributory

Anaemia
- Usually secondary to chronic inflammation
- May respond to iron supplements or misoprostol for blood loss induced by non-steroidal anti-inflammatory drugs

Chronic anterior uveitis
- Clinically silent and potentially blinding
- Patients at high risk have arthritis of pauciarticular onset before age of 6 and are positive for antinuclear antibodies
- Diagnosed by slit lamp examination—screening every 3–6 months is warranted for all patients with juvenile chronic arthritis except for those with systemic disease, those who are positive for rheumatoid factor, and those who have arthritis and enthesitis
- Treated with topical corticosteroids and mydriatics

Growth disturbance
- Localised—overgrowth (such as leg lengthening due to knee synovitis) or undergrowth (such as premature fusion of finger epiphyses)
- Generalised—growth failure secondary to severe inflammation or treatment with corticosteroids. Treatment with recombinant growth hormone improves growth rate in some cases

Amyloidosis
- Rare—results in proteinuria and hypoalbuminaemia
- May respond to chlorambucil

Joint failure
- About 5% of patients with juvenile chronic arthritis eventually require joint replacement
- Those at highest risk have polyarticular disease and are positive for rheumatoid factor

Early diagnosis and treatment by an experienced paediatric rheumatology team improves prognosis. The team should include experts in physiotherapy, occupational therapy, social work, nursing, splint making, and psychology. Ready access to orthopaedic surgery, dentistry and orthodontics, ophthalmology, psychiatry, and other paediatric specialties is also important. Treatment usually includes education about the disease, physical therapy, non-steroidal anti-inflammatory drugs, and intra-articular corticosteroids.

The progress of the disease must be monitored carefully. Clinical and laboratory evidence of disease activity should be assessed and recorded several times a year. Affected children rarely need hospitalisation, but it is indicated for inability to walk, progressive flexion deformities unresponsive to physiotherapy, and severe extra-articular features of disease (pericarditis, inanition, or anaemia). Physiotherapists, occupational therapists, clinic nurses, teachers, and other therapists should also be closely involved with monitoring disease. In particular, the range of motion of affected joints; the muscle bulk of affected limbs; and the physical, school, and social function of children should be formally recorded at least every six months.

Non-steroidal anti-inflammatory drugs

These are indicated in all children with active synovitis. Unless adverse effects are noted, each drug should be used for at least two to three months to ensure adequate time for a clinical response. The most common adverse effect is abdominal pain. This may be transient, but if it is not, misoprostal 10–20 µg/kg/day in divided doses seems to be effective. Other problems include changes in mood, rash (such as pseudoporphyria, described with naproxen), and, rarely, interstitial nephritis. Administration of more than one non-steroidal anti-inflammatory drug concurrently should be avoided owing to the additive risk of adverse effects. Discontinuation of these drugs may be considered if all clinical and laboratory features of the disease have been quiescent for six months or more.

Corticosteroids

Intra-articular corticosteroids are indicated for arthritis that is not controlled by non-steroidal anti-inflammatory drugs. Triamcinolone hexacetonide (0·5–1 mg/kg for each affected joint) is usually administered under sedation or general anaesthesia with aseptic "no touch" techniques. The maximum frequency of intra-articular treatment for individual joints is unknown but can be as often as every six months if there is a beneficial clinical response. Topical corticosteroids are the main treatment for chronic anterior uveitis. Oral or parenteral corticoisteroids may help to treat severe immobility, carditis, or severe anaemia but are otherwise best avoided because of their propensity for retarding growth and other adverse effects. The risk of osteopenia can be minimised with supplemental calcium (0·5–1 g/day) and vitamin D (calcitriol 0·25 mg/day). Deflazacort may be more "bone sparing" than prednisolone: it is slightly less potent (a dose of 6 mg of deflazacort is equivalent to 5 mg prednisolone) and should be widely available soon.

Differential diagnosis

Slowing acting antirheumatic drugs

These drugs are required for persistent active polyarthritis that is not controlled by non-steroidal anti-inflammatory drugs. Methotrexate helps up to 70% of patients: the starting dose of 0·3 mg/kg a week (taken orally) is increased at monthly intervals until clinical benefit is noted (up to a maximum dose of 1 mg/kg a week or 25 mg a week). Intramuscular or subcutaneous injections may improve the absorption of methotrexate in patients with non-responsive disease. Patients should be monitored every month for adverse effects including abnormalities in liver enzymes, bone marrow toxicity, mood changes, alteration of the urinary sediment, and ulceration of the mouth. There is little controlled scientific evidence to support the use of any other antirheumatic drugs in treating juvenile chronic arthritis, although results of open trials indicate that intramuscular gold may be effective. Sulphasalazine (50–60 mg/kg daily in divided doses) may also have a role in uncontrolled juvenile chronic arthritis, particularly for patients with arthritis and enthesitis that may be a precursor to ankylosing spondylitis.

Combination chemotherapy (such as methotrexate, intravenous methylprednisolone pulses, and cyclophosphamide) has been advocated for severe recalcitrant juvenile chronic arthritis of systemic onset. Intravenous gammaglobulin (doses of 1–2 g/kg) has also been used for juvenile chronic arthritis of systemic onset, but its efficacy was questionable in a recent controlled trial.

Immunisations

Very few patients with juvenile chronic arthritis are sufficiently immunosuppressed to warrant avoiding immunisations containing live viruses. Children with moderate to severe juvenile chronic arthritis often experience exacerbations of arthritis after influenza and other viral illnesses, and yearly influenza immunisation should be considered for these high risk children.

Many diseases may present with joint symptoms or have predominantly musculoskeletal features.

Mechanical disorders

Symptoms are usually related to physical activity and are more common in adolescents. They typically worsen during the day whereas inflammatory joint disease tends to be worse on awakening in the morning. The knee, ankle, hip, and back are most often affected, and associated conditions include localised and generalised hypermobility syndromes, developmental abnormalities such as osteochondritis, and structural disorders.

Non-accidental injury—Joint swelling from non-accidental injury may be due to traumatic periostitis, haemorrhage, or epiphyseal fracture. Any discrepancy between a patient's history and the physical findings should be carefully assessed. A radiographic skeletal survey and bone scan are indicated.

Inflammatory disorders

Reactive arthritis is one of the commonest causes of acute arthritis in children. It can be defined as an acute arthritis in the absence of intra-articular sepsis that occurs in close temporal association with an extra-articular infection. Rheumatic fever is now seen only rarely, and an isolated post-streptococcal arthritis is more common. Unlike in adults, in children the gastrointestinal tract is the commonest site of extra-articular infection (salmonella, yersinia, campylobacter, or shigella infections). Other forms of reactive arthritis reported in children include Lyme arthritis, mycoplasma arthritis, and illnesses after viral infections (influenza, rubella, coxsackie B, herpesvirus group, mumps, parvovirus B19, hepatitis B, and alphaviruses). Rarely, arthritis may precede other clinical features of infection, such as jaundice, but it more commonly follows the infection by one to three weeks.

Arthritis in children

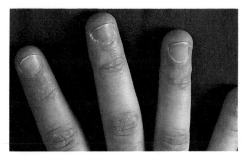

Gottron's papules in boy with juvenile dermatomyositis.

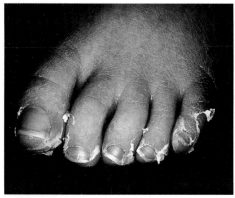

Desquamation of toes of child with Kawasaki disease.

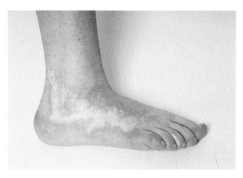

Localised scleroderma of the foot of an 11 year old girl.

The photograph of desquammation in Kawasaki disease was supplied by R G Levy, registrar in paediatrics, and B Bose-Haider, consultant paediatrician, from Fairfield Hospital, Bury.

Septic arthritis—Children with septic arthritis usually seem very unwell with high fever, a hot swollen joint, and severely restricted range of joint movement. Affected joints must be aspirated for diagnostic purposes before treatment is started. Patients should be treated with intravenous antibiotics for two to three weeks, followed by oral antibiotics until the erythrocyte sedimentation rate is normal and there are no clinical findings.

Systemic lupus erythematosus is rare in children. Unlike in adults, prominent presenting features in children include growth failure, constitutional disorders (fever, poor weight gain), and nephritis. Very rarely, transplacental transmission of maternal autoantibodies may result in a neonatal lupus syndrome characterised by congenital complete heart block, dermatitis, and cytopenia. In general, paediatric systemic lupus erythematosus is most severe during the first year after onset. The 15 year survival for children treated at major centres is 85–90%.

Juvenile dermatomyositis can be diagnosed by the combination of a progressive proximal myopathy and the typical dermatitis. Unlike adult dermatomyositis, it is not associated with an increased prevalence of neoplasia. Arthritis occurs in a third of cases. Life threatening complications include respiratory failure and aspiration. Joint contractures and soft tissue calcinosis may complicate the course of the disease. Concentrations of muscle enzymes (creatine phosphokinase, aspartate aminotransferase, lactate dehydrogenase) are commonly elevated, and serial monitoring is a valuable guide to disease activity. Electromyography and muscle biopsy should be reserved for the diagnosis of atypical cases. Muscle oedema can be quantified using magnetic resonance imaging, and this may be useful for monitoring and for guiding muscle biopsy.

Henoch-Schoenlein purpura—The combination of large joint arthritis, abdominal pain, and a purpuric rash over the lower legs and buttocks is sufficient to diagnose Henoch-Schoenlein purpura. It is the commonest vasculitis in childhood. The disease is usually transient, but about 3% of sufferers develop important nephritis and it is one of the commoner causes of chronic renal failure in children. Rarely, recurrent episodes of arthritis may occur.

Kawasaki disease is the second most common vasculitis in childhood and is probably underdiagnosed in Britain. The presence of at least five of six criteria is required for the diagnosis: prolonged spiking fever (>5 days), oral mucositis, polymorphous rash, cervical lymphadenopathy, conjunctivitis, and oedema followed by peeling of the extremities. Early diagnosis and treatment with intravenous gammaglobulin have substantially reduced the complication of coronary artery aneurysms. Arthritis is usually a transient feature of Kawasaki disease.

Scleroderma—Unlike in adults, scleroderma in children is usually localised. It may be associated with arthritis as part of a mixed connective tissue disorder.

Neoplasia

Arthritis may result from leukaemia, neuroblastoma, lymphoma, and, less often, from localised bone or joint related tumours. Very rarely, children with musculoskeletal symptoms may have a "preleukaemic" condition, the diagnosis only being confirmed months after the onset of symptoms. The commonest benign localised skeletal tumours of childhood are osteochondromas, chondromas, and osteoid osteomas. Fibrous cortical defects, bone cysts, and eosinophilic granulomas may cause diagnostic confusion with these lesions. Malignant bone tumours are rare, but those that occur in childhood include Ewing's sarcoma and osteosarcoma.

Idiopathic or stress associated conditions

The most dramatic musculoskeletal pains in young people are often associated with conditions which are not clearly inflammatory or mechanical. Emotional stress (overt or covert) is common in these patients and may arise from learning difficulties, overachievement, or non-accidental trauma. Associated features include easy fatiguability, poor attendance at school, pronounced limb or bodily dysfunction, and a non-restorative sleep pattern characterised by fatigue on awakening.

Sources of educational material about juvenile chronic arthritis

- The Children's Chronic Arthritis Association
  Telephone (01905) 763 556
- Young Arthritis Care
  Telephone (0171) 916 1500
- Arthritis and Rheumatism Council
  Telephone (01246) 558 033
  Handbooks available:
  When a young person has arthritis: a guide for teachers
  When your child has arthritis: a handbook for parents
- Academy Television
  Telephone (0113) 461 528
  Kids like us—A disease education video for patients with juvenile chronic arthritis

14 POLYMYALGIA RHEUMATICA AND GIANT CELL ARTERITIS

Gillian Pountain, Brian Hazleman

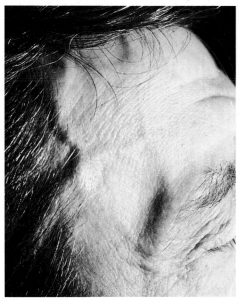

Swollen temporal artery of patient with giant cell arteritis.

In recent years giant cell arteritis and polymyalgia rheumatica have increasingly been considered as closely related conditions. The two syndromes form a spectrum of disease and affect the same types of patient. The conditions may occur independently or may occur in the same patient, either together or separated in time.

Polymyalgia rheumatica is a clinical syndrome of middle aged and elderly patients and is characterised by:

- Pain and stiffness in the neck and the shoulder and pelvic girdles
- Systemic features such as low grade fever, fatigue, and weight loss
- An increased erythrocyte sedimentation rate
- A dramatic response to small doses of corticosteroids.

Aetiology

Aetiology of polymyalgia rheumatica and giant cell arteritis

- There is often a distinct prodromal event resembling influenza, but results of viral studies are negative
- Lymphocytes in arteritic lesions express the T cell phenotype, and the CD4 subset predominates
- Frequency of HLA-DR4 is increased

Epidemiology of giant cell arteritis

- Peak incidence at ages 60–75
- Sex distribution of 3 women to 1 man
- Annual incidence 18/100 000 people aged over 50*
- Most reports from northern Europe and northern United States; mainly affects white people, but can occur worldwide
- Familial aggregation has been reported, suggesting genetic association

*Diagnosis confirmed by biopsy

Polymyalgia rheumatica—At present it is impossible to define the underlying pathological abnormality in polymyalgia rheumatica, and several different mechanisms may be responsible for a largely similar pattern of pain.

Giant cell arteritis is limited to vessels with an internal elastic component. Both humoral and cellular immunological mechanisms have been implicated in its development, and the latter seem to be more important.

Giant cell arteritis affects white people almost exclusively, but it has been reported in black Americans. In all studies both conditions are very rare under the age of 50 years. Reports from Olmsted County, Minnesota, and Gothenburg, Sweden, have shown that the incidence is increasing in women but not in men. About half of patients with giant cell arteritis have symptoms of polymyalgia rheumatica, whereas 15–50% of patients with polymyalgia rheumatica have giant cell arteritis. Problems with case definition and ascertainment complicate epidemiological observations.

Polymyalgia rheumatica and giant cell arteritis

Clinical features

Diagnosis may be difficult, and polymyalgia rheumatica is diagnosed by exclusion.

Polymyalgia rheumatica

Symptoms are usually bilateral and symmetrical. The predominant feature is usually stiffness that is particularly severe after rest and may prevent a patient getting out of bed. Affected structures feel tender, and shoulder movement may be restricted if diagnosis is delayed. Muscular pain is often diffuse and is accentuated by movement. Muscle strength is unimpaired, but the pain makes interpretation of muscle testing difficult. Persistent synovitis is uncommon and suggests an alternative diagnosis such as rheumatoid arthritis.

Giant cell arteritis

This condition causes a wide range of symptoms, but most patients have clinical features related to affected arteries. Common features include fatigue, headaches, joint pain, and tenderness of the scalp, particularly around the temporal and occipital arteries. The arteries are thickened, tender, and nodular, with pulsation being absent or reduced. Visual symptoms may take the form of amaurosis fugax, diplopia, and partial or complete loss of vision.

Differential diagnosis of polymyalgia rheumatica

Myeloma
Neoplastic disease
Joint disease
Osteoarthritis, particularly of cervical spine
Rheumatoid arthritis
Connective tissue disease
Muscle disease
Polymyositis
Myopathy
Infections

Investigations

Baseline investigations to aid diagnosis

The erythrocyte sedimentation rate and concentration of C reactive protein are usually, but not necessarily, raised in the two conditions: there are many case reports of giant cell arteritis proved by biopsy with normal or slightly increased erythrocyte sedimentation rates. Repeated measurements may show raised erythrocyte sedimentation rates after an initial normal value.

Patients may have normocytic anaemia, and the concentration of hepatic alkaline phosphatase is often raised. These features, together with the clinical picture of weight loss, may resemble those of occult malignancy.

If polymyalgia rheumatica is suspected other conditions must be excluded by appropriate investigations.

Investigations at presentation of polymyalgia rheumatica and giant cell arteritis

Polymyalgia rheumatica
- Erythrocyte sedimentation rate
- Acute phase proteins
- Full blood count
- Biochemical profile
- Protein electrophoresis
- Bence Jones proteins
- Thyroid function
- Chest radiograph
- Rheumatoid factor
- Muscle enzymes (if indicated)

Giant cell arteritis
- Erythrocyte sedimentation rate
- C reactive protein
- Full blood count
- Liver function tests
- Consider temporal artery biopsy

Biopsy

Some patients with polymyalgia rheumatica but without symptoms of giant cell arteritis have positive results from temporal artery biopsies. Thus, all suspected cases of polymyalgia rheumatica or giant cell arteritis might benefit from temporal artery biopsy. However, the problems of obtaining biopsies rapidly make this impractical. The choice of patients for biopsy depends on local circumstances, but a pragmatic policy would be to select only patients with suspected giant cell arteritis (not those with obvious clinical features). Patients with pure polymyalgia rheumatica would need to be monitored carefully for development of clinical giant cell arteritis.

A third of patients with signs and symptoms of cranial arteritis may have negative temporal artery biopsies, which may be due to the localised involvement of arteries in the head and neck. After one week of corticosteroid treatment the chance of obtaining a positive biopsy result is only 10%, so biopsy is worthwhile only in the first few days of treatment. However, treatment for suspected giant cell arteritis should not be delayed simply to allow a biopsy to be carried out.

Biopsy for giant cell arteritis

- Perform biopsy if diagnosis is in doubt, particularly if systemic symptoms predominate
- Biopsy is most useful within 24 hours of starting treatment, but do not delay treatment for sake of biopsy
- A negative result does not exclude giant cell arteritis
- A positive result helps to prevent later doubts about diagnosis, particularly if treatment causes complications

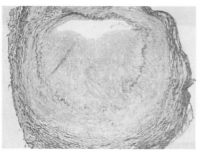 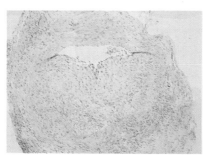

Histological appearance of artery affected by giant cell arteritis: decreased lumen and disruption of internal elastic lamina (left); inflammatory cell infiltrate (right).

Histology of giant cell arteritis

Giant cell arteritis is one of the most distinctive pathological disorders. In the acute phase the histological changes are characteristic, but several arterial diseases with different clinical syndromes may also have a granulomatous histological appearance. Typical changes include a giant cell infiltrate and disruption of the media and internal elastic lamina. The intima is thickened and oedematous, and the lumen is restricted.

Pathologists should be aware of the wide range of histological changes that occur as part of normal aging and must not interpret these as evidence of healed arteritis. The histological changes of healed arteritis include medial chronic inflammation with a growth of new blood vessels, focal medial scarring, and intimal fibrosis.

Treatment

Treatment of polymyalgia rheumatica and giant cell arteritis*

Polymyalgia rheumatica

Initial dose—Prednisolone 10–20 mg daily for one month

Reduce dose by 2·5 mg every 2–4 weeks until dose is 10 mg, then by 1 mg every 4–6 weeks (or until symptoms return)

Maintenance dose of about 10 mg by six months after start of treatment and 5–7·5 mg by one year. Most patients require treatment for 3–4 years but withdrawal after two years is worth attempting

Giant cell arteritis

Initial dose—Prednisolone 20–40 mg daily for eight weeks. Patients with ocular symptoms may need up to 80 mg daily

Reduce dose by 5 mg every 3–4 weeks until dose is 10 mg daily, then as for polymyalgia rheumatica

Maintenance dose of about 3 mg daily may be required

*Recurrence of symptoms requires an increase in prednisolone dose

---

Diagnosing relapse of polymyalgia rheumatica and giant cell arteritis

- Principally a clinical diagnosis
- Erythrocyte sedimentation rate and concentration of C reactive protein are often not raised in relapses; when they are raised another cause is often found

---

Risks of side effects from corticosteroid treatment

- Increased risk with high initial doses (>30 mg) of prednisolone, maintenance doses of 10 mg, and high cumulative dosages
- Maintenance doses of 5 mg prednisolone are relatively safe

Treatment with corticosteroids is mandatory for giant cell arteritis to prevent vascular complications, particularly blindness, as well as for rapidly relieving symptoms: before corticosteroids were used the reported prevalence of blindness was 30–60%. Corticosteroids are usually also used for polymyalgia rheumatica because of the possibility of blindness.

Most patients require three to four years of treatment with corticosteroids, and many need continued treatment with small doses. If a patient needs high doses of corticosteroid, azathioprine or methotrexate can be used to reduce the required dose by their corticosteroid sparing effect, but regular monitoring of blood count and testing of liver function are required.

Relapses

Relapses are most likely in the first 18 months of treatment, but they can occur after apparently successful treatment when corticosteroids have been discontinued. At present there is no way of predicting which patients are most at risk. Diagnosis of relapse should be made on clinical features since the erythrocyte sedimentation rate and concentration of C reactive protein are often not raised during relapses or may be increased due to other causes.

During relapses the dose of prednisolone should be increased to the dose given before relapse or more, depending on the severity of symptoms.

Complications

Patients are at risk of the usual side effects of corticosteroids. The reported incidence of side effects ranges from 20% to 50%. In one study side effects were significantly more common with a starting dose of prednisolone of 30 mg or more or a mean maintenance dose of over 5 mg. Side effects can be minimised by using low doses of prednisolone whenever possible and giving corticosteroid sparing drugs such as azathioprine and methotrexate when necessary.

In elderly people corticosteroid treatment carries the risk of increasing osteoporosis. For women, disodium etidronate with calcium carbonate is the most effective prophylaxis. It increases the spinal bone mineral density of patients taking corticosteroids by about 4% after one year and by 4.8% after two years.[1]

1 Skingle SJ, Crisp AJ. Increased bone density in patients on steroids with etidronate. *Lancet* 1994;**344**:543–4.

15 SYSTEMIC LUPUS ERYTHEMATOSUS AND LUPUS-LIKE SYNDROMES

Elaine M Hay, Michael L Snaith

Classification criteria for systemic lupus erythematosus (revised 1982[1])

To be classified as having systemic lupus erythematosus, patients must have at least four of the following criteria in the course of their disease:

- Malar disease
- Photosensitivity
- Arthritis
- Renal disorder
- Haematological disorder
- Presence of anti-nuclear antibodies (ANA)
- Discoid rash
- Oral ulcers
- Serositis
- Neurological disorder
- Immunological disorder

Systemic lupus erythematosus is one of a family of interrelated and overlapping autoimmune rheumatic disorders that includes rheumatoid arthritis, scleroderma, polymyositis, dermatomyositis, and Sjögren's syndrome. The disease can present as a wide variety of clinical features, reflecting the many organ systems that can be affected. This clinical diversity is matched serologically by a wide spectrum of autoantibodies, which tend to cluster in relation to the clinical pattern.

Systemic lupus erythematosus is rare: a general practice with 10 000 registered patients is unlikely to have more than three or four patients with the disease at any one time. It is nine times more common in women than in men, and nine times more common in Afro-Caribbeans and Asians than in white patients. Thus, general practitioners' experience will vary greatly according to the ethnic mix of their registered population.

(F:M 9:1)

Clinical presentation

Consider systemic lupus erythematosus in a young woman presenting with "seronegative rheumatoid arthritis"

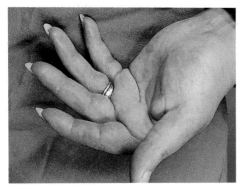

Jaccoud-type arthropathy; non-erosive deformity of fingers owing to tendons being affected.

Because lupus is so uncommon, one difficulty is considering the possibility in the first place, particularly if the presentation is atypical or the patient is elderly or male. Differentiating lupus from similar disorders can be difficult, particularly early in the course of the disease, because many of the clinical features are common non-specific complaints. Although classification criteria for lupus are widely accepted, they are more appropriate for classifying patients in clinical trials or epidemiological studies than for making a diagnosis in individual patients. Lupus should be considered when characteristic clinical features—most commonly arthralgia, mucocutaneous manifestations, and fatigue—occur in combination or evolve over time.

Arthralgia

Generalised arthralgia, with pronounced morning stiffness but little to find on examination, is characteristic, and pain may be considerable. Although symptoms may mimic early rheumatoid arthritis, joint swelling (synovitis) is much less noticeable. About 20% of patients will develop deformity (Jaccoud-type arthropathy) of the hands owing to tendons being affected. This is reversible in its early stages, but it can become permanent and joint instability may require surgery.

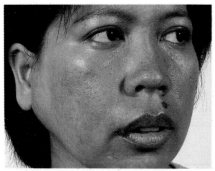

Classic malar "butterfly" rash of systemic lupus erythematosus after exposure to sunlight (reproduced with patient's permission).

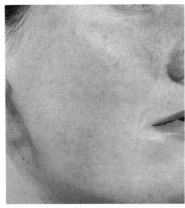

Parvovirus "slapped cheek" rash.

Mucocutaneous manifestations

A wide variety of manifestations is possible. The classic malar "butterfly" rash is the textbook presentation; it usually presents abruptly after exposure to sunlight and lasts for several days or weeks. However, most facial rashes presenting in primary care are not caused by lupus. More common causes include acne rosacea and the parvovirus "slapped cheek" rash.

Rapid hair loss can be a useful marker of active disease and can lead to alopecia. The hair will, however, regrow when the disease remits unless the scalp is scarred. Ulceration of the mouth or, less commonly, the nose or vagina may or may not be painful, but it is also usually self limiting. Raynaud's phenomenon occurs in about half of patients at presentation, but it is less common and usually milder than with scleroderma or related syndromes. Conversely, most patients who present to their general practitioner with Raynaud's syndrome will not have systemic lupus erythematosus. If they are positive for antinuclear antibodies they are likely to eventually develop a connective tissue disease.

Fatigue

Severe fatigue in conjunction with some of the above symptoms may reflect a flare up of the disease. Chronic fatigue, however, is almost invariable in established systemic lupus erythematosus and may reflect underlying depression or cardiovascular deconditioning.

Major organ disease

Patients greatly fear developing diseases of major organs such as the kidneys or central nervous system. Reassuringly, these do not occur in most patients, and when they do they are usually a relatively early feature. Nevertheless, they are potentially life threatening and are associated with a poorer prognosis overall.

Renal disease occurs in 20–50% of all patients at some time during their disease, but end stage renal failure is rare (<5%). The start of disease may be insidious, and patients should therefore have regular dipstick testing of their urine for protein to facilitate early and aggressive treatment.

"Cerebral lupus" is probably overdiagnosed. For example, anxiety and depression are common but are usually caused by psychological stresses associated with a painful, unpredictable, chronic illness rather than reflecting cerebral lupus. Management should focus on personal social problems such as isolation or marital stress. Headaches have a wide variety of possible causes. "Tension headache" can be difficult to distinguish from "lupus headache"—both may be unremitting and unresponsive to simple analgesics. The latter is extremely uncommon, however, and is usually associated with other features of active disease. Migraine is more common in patients with lupus than in the general population, particularly in patients with antiphospholipid antibodies.

Cardiopulmonary disease—Pleurisy and pericarditis may be presenting features, and pleuritic pain may mimic that of infection or embolism. Although lung disease is uncommon, it is difficult to treat.

Factors that increase probability of associated connective tissue disease in patients with Raynaud's phenomenon

- Onset of condition in childhood or old age
- Asymmetrical manifestation of symptoms
- Severe disease threatening viability of peripheries
- Associated with other symptoms such as arthralgia, fatigue, rash, etc
- Associated with abnormal results of blood tests (such as raised erythrocyte sedimentation rate, anaemia, presence of antinuclear antibodies)

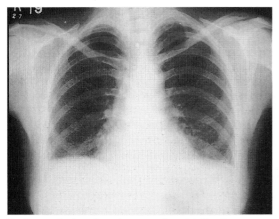

Radiograph showing changes of restrictive lung disease in patient with lupus—"shrinking lung" appearance and linear shadows. Pulmonary function tests may eventually stabilise, but pulmonary hypertension occasionally develops.

Investigations

Blood tests are useful for confirming the diagnosis of systemic lupus erythematosus and for differentiating between various subsets of the disease but are less useful for monitoring disease activity. The most useful screening tests are a complete blood count, erythrocyte sedimentation rate, and testing for antinuclear antibody.

There is often a normochromic normocytic anaemia when the disease is active. Leucopenia or lymphocytopenia is common and is useful for differentiating between systemic lupus erythematosus and rheumatoid arthritis. Thrombocytopenia is an uncommon but well recognised complication of lupus. Measuring C reactive protein can be a useful test for distinguishing between a lupus flare and infection: it usually remains normal in a flare, unless accompanied by serositis or synovitis, but is elevated in infection. The erythrocyte sedimentation rate will be elevated in both and occasionally remains considerably elevated when the disease seems to be clinically quiescent.

The erythrocyte sedimentation rate should not be relied on to dictate treatment decisions

---

If the test for antinuclear antibodies is negative, systemic lupus erythematosus is extremely unlikely

---

Systemic lupus erythematosus and lupus-like syndromes

More than 95% of patients with systemic lupus erythematosus have antinuclear antibodies. However, such antibodies may be found in other autoimmune disorders and (in low concentration) in chronic infection and elderly people. Fewer than half of patients with lupus have antibodies to double stranded DNA at presentation: thus it is not a good screening test. However, rising titres of these antibodies, particularly if accompanied by falling concentrations of C3 and C4, may herald the start of renal disease. C3 and C4 are insensitive diagnostically. Antibodies to soluble cellular antigens (such as La, Ro, U1 RNP, and Jo-1) can be useful for distinguishing between lupus subsets.[2][3] Antiphospholipid antibodies (such as anticardiolipin antibodies or lupus anticoagulant) identify a subset of patients at particular risk of thromboembolic complications or fetal loss.

Management

Firstly, patients need explanation and reassurance, as the liability to episodic flare engenders insecurity and apprehension. It should be emphasised that serious complications are rare and that most patients have a normal life expectancy.

Preventing lupus flares

Patients should avoid exposure to sunlight (including sunbeds), which, as well as precipitating acute or subacute skin lesions, may also cause a generalised lupus flare. Sunscreens with a high protection factor (factor 15 or higher) effective against ultraviolet A and B should be applied liberally, and long sleeved clothes and sunhats should be worn in sunny weather. Topical corticosteroid preparations are sometimes helpful for chronic skin lesions but should be used sparingly to avoid thinning of the skin.

Oral contraceptive pills containing low doses of oestrogen are probably safe with mild lupus but should be used with caution by patient with severe lupus since they can theoretically cause a flare. They are contraindicated in patients with migraine, hypertension, a history of thrombosis, or high titres of anticardiolipin antibodies. Progestogen-only oral contraceptives are safe. Intrauterine devices should be avoided if possible because of an increased risk of infection. The evidence for use of hormone replacement therapy is not yet clear enough to be able to give general advice: probably the best policy is cautious introduction of low dose oestrogen when the disease is quiescent with closer than usual monitoring.

Differentiating between a lupus flare and infection can be difficult. Infection is an important cause of mortality in patients with systemic lupus erythematosus, particularly in those taking corticosteroids or immunosuppressive drugs. Furthermore, intercurrent infection can precipitate a lupus flare. Hence it is important to maintain a high index of suspicion and regard any flu-like or feverish episode lasting more than a day or two as infection unless proved otherwise. Sulphonamides should usually be avoided because they may cause rash or sudden profound neutropenia.

Symptomatic and supportive treatment

Most common symptoms of systemic lupus erythematosus can be safely treated symptomatically. Arthralgia, headaches, and non-specific chest pains may be helped by non-steroidal anti-inflammatory drugs or simple analgesics. Blood pressure should be checked regularly and hypertension treated intensively, particularly if there is renal disease.

Corticosteroid treatment for a severe lupus flare

Continuous oral treatment
Starting dose of prednisolone is usually
   0·75–1 mg/kg
Treatment continued at same dose for
   4–10 weeks depending on clinical response
Careful reduction can then be attempted

Intravenous pulses
Methylprednisolone 0·5–1·5 g repeated
   1–3 times
Suppresses symptoms and may modify
   outcome, but avascular necrosis remains a
   risk

Intramuscular or oral minipulses
Such as 100–125 mg prednisolone acetate
   intramuscularly
Safer and cheaper than and probably as
   effective as other methods for symptomatic
   relief

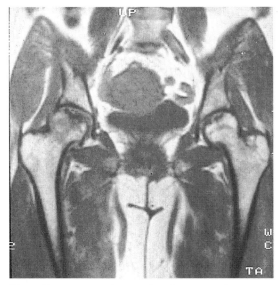

Magnetic resonance image showing avascular necrosis of hips. Avascular necrosis may affect any joint, and treatment with high dose corticosteroid is a particular risk factor.

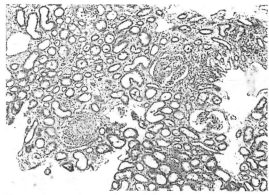

Severe lupus glomerulonephritis: appearance confirms end stage renal failure with glomerular loss. Continued treatment with immunosuppressive drugs and high dose corticosteroids is unlikely to achieve any improvement in function and would probably result only in further toxicity. (With less histological change, further immunosuppression might be justified to delay need for dialysis).

Disease modifying drugs

Corticosteroids have transformed the outlook for patients with lupus but at a considerable price: much of the increased mortality late in the course of the disease (due to infection, cardiovascular disease, or fracture complications) may be attributable to these drugs. Once an acute episode is under control the dose of corticosteroid should be slowly reduced; complete withdrawal is optimal, but many patients are best managed with a small maintenance dose of perhaps 5 mg or less a day. The dose of prednisolone should not be increased for non-specific constitutional symptoms in the absence of corroborative physical signs or abnormal laboratory results, even though this may make the patient feel better. Few lupus complications require immediate corticosteroid treatment—it is often best to wait and see for a day or two to avoid frequent increases in dose for non-specific symptoms. Arthralgia in systemic lupus erythematosus responds poorly to low dose prednisolone and usually does not warrant a high dose.

Antimalarial drugs—Chloroquine phosphate (250 mg daily or alternate days) or hydroxychloroquine (200–400 mg daily) is the mainstay of treatment for skin or joint disorders. At these doses ocular complications are extremely rare, but it is prudent to use the lowest effective dose. Rheumatologists and ophthalmologists continue to disagree about the need for routine screening. Hydroxychloroquine may be safer, though more expensive, than chloroquine. The total dose of chloroquine should not exceed 300 g, but it is not clear whether there should be such a limit for hydroxychloroquine.

Immunosuppressive drugs—Azathioprine, methotrexate, and cyclophosphamide are generally reserved for life threatening diseases of major organs such as the kidneys. They should be instituted and monitored at specialist centres, with appropriate counselling given about the short and long term side effects. Cyclophosphamide, whether continuous oral, pulse, or intravenous, is of proved benefit in treating renal lupus but is often associated with side effects that can be severe (such as infertility, premature menopause, or bladder cancer). Gamete storage should be offered before start of treatment when possible. Mesna may be used to reduce the risk of bladder toxicity with intravenous treatment, but oral mesna is not feasible for patients receiving continuous oral treatment. All these immunosuppressive drugs have the potential to suppress bone marrow activity, and frequent checks of complete blood count and differential white cell count are mandatory.

Outcome with systemic lupus erythematosus

Early studies reported that fewer than half of patients survived five years after diagnosis, but this figure has steadily improved. Recent studies report five year survival rates of 86–88% and 10 year survival rates of 76–87%. Patients who are non-white, male, or at the extremes of the age range fare worst. Most patients with lupus die from causes unrelated to the disease, but deaths (such as those due to infection or ischaemic heart disease) are increasingly related to treatment. Renal replacement therapy ensures that death from renal failure is uncommon.

Pregnancy with systemic lupus erythematosus

There is no evidence for reduced fertility in patients with systemic lupus erythematosus, and pregnancy presents little hazard for the mother if the lupus is mild or stable. Pre-existing renal disease may, however, worsen during pregnancy, and complications such as hypertension may be more difficult to control. Pre-eclamptic toxaemia may be difficult to distinguish from renal flare.

There is an increased rate of fetal loss, particularly during the second trimester, in patients with high titres of antiphospholipid antibodies. Pregnancies in such women should be monitored carefully in specialist units. Overall, there is no increased risk of fetal abnormalities, but drug treatment during pregnancy may pose problems. Antimetabolites are contraindicated because of teratogenesis, but low dose prednisolone, chloroquine, and azathioprine are probably safe.

Lupus-like syndromes

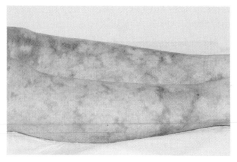

Livedo reticularis in patient with antiphospholipid syndrome.

Drugs implicated in causing lupus-like syndromes

Common
- Hydralazine
- Procainamide
- Anticonvulsants (phenytoin, hydantoins, primidone)
- Isoniazid

Rare
- Chlorpromazine
- Penicillamine
- Practolol
- Antithyroid drugs (propylthiouracil, methylthiouracil)
- Methyldopa

Clinical features of overlap syndromes

- Raynaud's phenomenon
- "Sausage" digits
- Periungual vascular distortion
- Hyperglobulinaemia and presence of antibodies to several soluble nuclear and cytoplasmic antigens
- Relative lack of cerebritis, antibodies to DNA, and immune complex glomerulonephritis
- Eventual outcome of cardiopulmonary disease

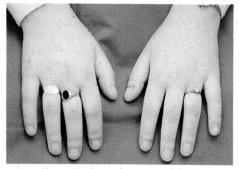

Sausage fingers of patient with mixed connective tissue disease.

Antiphospholipid syndrome

This may occur in patients with coexisting systemic lupus erythematosus or occur alone (primary antiphospholipid syndrome). It is characterised by thrombosis, livedo reticularis, and sometimes thrombocytopenia together with the lupus anticoagulant or antiphospholipid antibodies.

Subacute cutaneous lupus erythematosus

Intense photosensitivity and antibodies to La and Ro are the essential features of this relatively rare syndrome.

Discoid lupus erythematosus

In this condition lesions are obviously discoid, systemic features are rare and mild, and autoantibodies are low in titre.

Incipient lupus

Some patients do not progress to very active disease, and their condition is characterised by mild arthralgia, rashes, or serositis with weak positivity for antinuclear antibodies.

Neonatal lupus syndrome

A small proportion of babies born to mothers with systemic lupus erythematosus (which is often mild and may even have been unrecognised) develop the neonatal lupus syndrome. This syndrome appears to be restricted to babies whose mothers have antibodies to Ro (SS-A) or La (SS-B) antigens. A self limiting skin rash, which may be severe, is the most common presentation. Rarely, babies may have permanent heart block secondary to a conduction defect, which may require treatment with a cardiac pacemaker.

Drug induced lupus

Lupus-like syndromes may occasionally be induced by some drugs. They mostly consist of arthralgia with positivity for antinuclear antibodies, and renal disease is rare. Antibodies to DNA are rare, but antihistone antibodies are characteristic. The syndrome usually resolve when the offending drug is withdrawn, but antinuclear antibodies persist for months after.

Overlap syndromes

It has been suggested that the only true lupus syndrome consists of nephritis, photosensitivity, serositis, and antibodies to DNA. While this might be too purist a view, it is often difficult to categorise patients; criteria such as those for systemic lupus erythematosus[1] or those suggested for mixed connective tissue disease[4] do not cover all situations. Convention, however, prefers some form of categorisation, and the syndromes usually termed "overlap" (though some prefer the term undifferentiated connective tissue disease) tend to have certain characteristic features. Patients also prefer their doctor to be able to attach a label to their condition that is acceptable to others and carries some certainty with regard to prognosis and management.

Prognosis is on a case by case basis, depending on the rate of progression and severity and nature of involvement of organ systems. Management is similar in principle to that for systemic lupus erythematosus: the pattern of involvement dictating the treatment. It is clear that mixed connective tissue disease, for example, is not a robust syndrome; clinical expression tends to focus on a scleroderma-like, rheumatoid-like, or myositis-like syndrome, often with cardiopulmonary features dictating the outcome.

1 Tan EM, Cohen ES, Fries JF, Masi AT, McShane DJ, Rothfield NF, *et al*. The 1982 revised criteria for the classification of systemic lupus erythematosus. *Arthritis Rheum* 1982;25:1271–7.
2 Maddison PJ. Autoantibody profile. *Oxford textbook of rheumatology*. Vol 1. Oxford: Oxford University Press, 1993:389–96.
3 Isenberg DA, Horsfall AC. Systemic lupus erythematosus. *Oxford textook of rheumatology*. Vol 2. Oxford: Oxford University Press, 1993:733–55.
4 Alarcon-Segovia D, Cardiel MM. Comparison between 3 diagnostic criteria for mixed connective tissue disease: a study of 593 patients. *J Rheumatol* 1989;16:328–34.

16 RAYNAUD'S PHENOMENON, SCLERODERMA, AND OVERLAP SYNDROMES

David A Isenberg, Carol Black

Raynaud's phenomenon

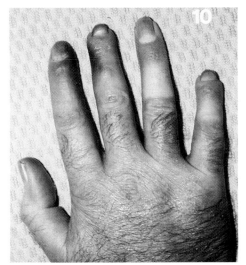

Well defined blanching of skin characteristic of Raynaud's phenomenon.

Several rheumatological conditions are linked to impaired peripheral circulation. These abnormalities may take various forms, including chilblains, acrocyanosis, and Raynaud's phenomenon. This last condition, described by the French clinician Maurice Raynaud in 1862, occurs in up to 5% of an otherwise healthy population, but may be a link between certain autoimmune rheumatic diseases. Raynaud's disease refers to the development of trophic changes as a result of microcirculatory damage and prolonged local ischaemia. Fortunately, gangrene is relatively rare, and, because patients are often young, recovery may be remarkable.

Disturbances of peripheral circulatory system

Chilblains—Painful, burning, or itching erythematosus lesions of hands or feet (rarely ulceration) precipitated by damp and cold (especially if inadequate clothing worn)

Acrocyanosis—Persistent cold, blue, and rather sweaty appearance, usually of hands

Raynaud's phenomenon—Episodic, clearly demarcated two or three phase colour change—white (ischaemia), then often blue (stasis), then red (reactive hyperaemia)—of fingers and sometimes toes (rarely nose, tongue, or ears) in response to cold or, less often, emotion

---

Raynaud's phenomenon as a predictor of autoimmune rheumatic disease

Over 90% of patients with Raynaud's phenomenon are female and, at the time of presentation, are often aged under 25. Up to 5% of patients presenting with the condition eventually develop an autoimmune rheumatic disease. The presence of abnormal nail fold capillaries (detected by capillaroscopy) and antinuclear antibodies are of particular value in predicting this development.

Prevalence of Raynaud's phenomenon in autoimmune rheumatic diseases

Rheumatoid arthritis	<5%
Systemic lupus erythematosus	20–30%
Sjögrens syndrome	20–30%
Myositis	25%
Scleroderma	>95%

Points to consider when looking for underlying cause of Raynaud's phenomenon

- Occupation—working outdoors, using vibrating tools, exposure to chemicals such as vinyl chloride
- Examination of peripheral and central vascular system for proximal vascular occlusion
- Drugs—such as β blockers, ergotamines, oral contraceptives, bleomycin
- Symptoms of other connective tissue disorders:
  Arthralgia or arthritis Alopecia Skin rashes
  Cerebral symptoms Photosensitivity Dry eyes or mouth
  Mouth ulcers Muscle weakness Respiratory or cardiac problems

---

Investigations of patients with Raynaud's phenomenon to test for autoimmune rheumatic disease

- Full blood count and erythrocyte sedimentation rate
- Total immunoglobulin and electrophoresis strip
- Urine analysis
- Nail fold capillaroscopy
- Chest x rays
- Renal and liver function tests
- Test for antinuclear antibody
- Hand x rays

Primary and secondary Raynaud's phenomenon are distinguished by a combination of clinical examination and laboratory investigations. Physical examination should include assessment of peripheral pulses, measurement of blood pressure in both arms, and examination of the neck for the tenderness often associated with a cervical rib. A negative test for antinuclear antibody in an otherwise healthy patient is reassuring but does not completely exclude subsequent development of an autoimmune rheumatic disease. Different types of antinuclear antibody may be specific for certain diseases and so may help in diagnosis. Plethysmography, Doppler ultrasonography, and laser Doppler flowmetry with direct capillaroscopy and thermal entrainment have been used to measure vascular phenomena objectively.

Patient support organisations

The Raynaud's and Scleroderma Association Trust
- 112 Crewe Road, Alsager, Cheshire ST7 25A
  Telephone (01270) 872776

The Scleroderma Society
- 61 Sandpit Lane, St Albans, Hertfordshire AL1 4EY
  Telephone (01727) 55054

Drugs for treating Raynaud's phenomenon

- Nifedipine (Adalat Retard 20 mg daily)
- Diltiazem hydrochloride 60 mg thrice daily
- Nicardipine hydrochloride 20 mg thrice daily
- Felodipine 5–10 mg daily
- Isradipine 1 mg twice daily, increasing to 2 mg twice daily after four weeks if necessary
- Concentrated fish oils (Maxepa 5 capsules twice daily)
- Gamolenic acid (Epogam 4–6 capsules twice daily)
- Captopril 6·25 mg daily, increasing to 18·75 mg or 25 mg daily if necessary

Management

Raynaud's phenomenon can be helped by general measures, most importantly by stopping smoking. Patients should also avoid known exacerbating factors such as exposure to cold (patients should wear very warm gloves and socks) and use of vibrating tools. A variety of warming devices such as electrically heated gloves are available, and relevant information can be obtained from patient support organisations.

Some patients with primary Raynaud's phenomenon and most with the condition secondary to an underlying autoimmune rheumatic disease require drug treatment. Nifedipine, a calcium channel blocker, is often helpful. The modified release preparation is preferable as it reduces the common side effects of headache and flushing, which are due to central as well as peripheral vasodilatation. Other calcium channel blockers and angiotensin converting enzyme inhibitors may also help. Some patients have noted an improvement after changing to diets supplemented with fish oils.

When tissue nutrition is compromised with ulceration or gangrene intravenous vasodilatation is essential. Prostacyclin infusions, starting with about 5 µg/kg/hour, can be increased to 15 µg/kg/hour if patients can tolerate the side effects, which include flushing and headache. These infusions are usually given over five hour periods on several successive days, but continuous infusions have been given for impending gangrene. Calcitonin gene related peptide, a very powerful vasodilator, is currently under trial, with some success. Digital sympathectomy may also be of value.

Scleroderma (systemic sclerosis)

Characteristic findings and suggested treatment for limited cutaneous scleroderma

Early stage (≤ 10 years after onset)
Constitutional symptoms—None
Skin thickening—No or minimal progression
Organs affected—Raynaud's phenomenon, ulcers of digital tips, oesophageal symptoms
Treatment—Vascular treatment (oral or intravenous) with or without digital sympathectomy, removal of calcinosis, treat oesophageal problems

Late stage (> 10 years after onset)
Constitutional symptoms—Secondary to complications below
Skin thickening—Stable
Organs affected—Raynaud's phenomenon, ulcers of digital tips, calcinosis, oesophageal stricture, small bowel malabsorption, pulmonary hypertension
Treatment—Vascular treatment (oral or intravenous) with or without digital sympathectomy, removal of calcinosis, treat oesophageal and midgut problems

The term scleroderma encompasses a spectrum of disorders that includes localised scleroderma (morphea), which mainly causes dermal fibrosis; juvenile scleroderma, which is usually localised but can present with systemic disease; and scleroderma-like disorders. The diagnosis of scleroderma should be doubted in the absence of Raynaud's phenomenon. There are two main subsets of scleroderma according to the duration of Raynaud's phenomenon before the start of symptoms and signs suggestive of scleroderma.

Limited cutaneous scleroderma

Patients who develop this condition (previously called CREST) may have Raynaud's phenomenon for years before the appearance of the condition's characteristic symptoms: calcium deposits in the skin, painful digital scars and ulcers, dilated blood vessels (telangiectasia), and oesophageal dysmotility and reflux. There are few if any constitutional symptoms, and skin fibrosis is often restricted to sclerodactyly and microstomia, with minimal progression. Raynaud's phenomenon, pitting scars, digital ulcers, and telangiectasia can all be troublesome, and oesophageal symptoms are common. Patients may not be aware of the thickening of their fingers, but unsightly puckering, wrinkling and tightening of the skin around the mouth are soon noticed.

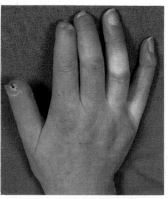 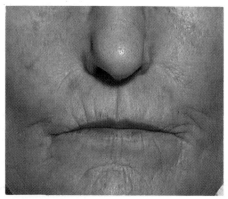

Characteristic features of limited cutaneous scleroderma: (left) puffy fingers, tight skin, Raynaud's phenomenon, loss of distal digits, and ulceration of tips of digits; (right) microstomia and telangiectasia.

Characteristic findings and suggested treatment for diffuse cutaneous scleroderma

Early stage (≤5 years after onset)

Constitutional symptoms—Fatigue, weight loss

Skin thickening—Rapid progression

Organs affected—Risk of renal, cardiac, pulmonary (fibrosis), gastrointestinal, articular, and muscular damage

Treatment—Immunosuppression, antifibrotic treatment, vasodilation, physiotherapy, and occupational therapy as appropriate

Late stage (>5 years after onset)

Constitutional symptoms—None

Skin thickening—Stable or regression

Organs affected—Musculoskeletal deformities, progression of existing visceral diseases but reduced risk of new conditions

Treatment—Treat complications, reduce antifibrotic treatment, continue vascular treatment

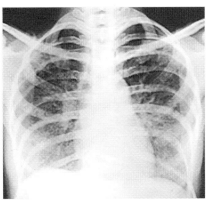

Chest radiograph of diffuse interstitial lung disease in patient with scleroderma.

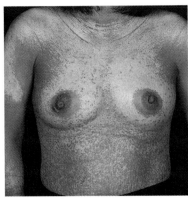

Hypopigmentation caused by diffuse cutaneous scleroderma.

Subsets of scleroderma

Limited cutaneous scleroderma
- Raynaud's phenomenon for years (sometimes decades) before start of scleroderma
- Skin is affected only at the extremities (hands, face, feet, and forearms) or is not affected
- Substantial proportion of patients develop pulmonary hypertension of late onset (after 10–15 years) with or without interstitial lung disease, skin calcifications, telangiectasia, and gastrointestinal symptoms
- High prevalence of anticentromere antibodies (70–80%)
- Dilated capillary loops of nail folds, usually without capillary dropout

Diffuse cutaneous scleroderma
- Start of skin changes (puffy or hidebound) within one year of start of Raynaud's phenomenon
- Skin of trunk and extremities affected
- Presence of tendon friction rubs
- Substantial proportion of patients have early onset of interstitial lung disease, oliguric renal failure, diffuse gastointestinal disease, and myocardial disease
- Dilated capillaries of nail fold and capillary dropout
- Antibodies to scleroderma-70 (topoisomerase-1) in 30% of patients

"Scleroderma sine scleroderma"
- Raynaud's phenomenon may or may not be present
- Skin not affected
- Presents with pulmonary fibrosis, scleroderma renal crisis, cardiac disease, and gastrointestinal disease
- Antinuclear antibodies (scleroderma-70, anticentromere, and antinucleolar antibodies) may be present

In the last stage of this condition the vascular disease often worsens, with widespread telangiectasia, ulcers and calcinosis, and pulmonary hypertension. Pulmonary interstitial disease may occur as a late complication. Visceral symptoms can worsen, with development of oesophageal strictures, small bowel disease, malabsorption, pseudo-obstruction, and anal incontinence. About half of all patients with scleroderma have the anticentromere antibody, but it is much more common with limited cutaneous scleroderma.

Diffuse cutaneous scleroderma

Patients destined to develop this condition often have a short history and abrupt onset of Raynaud's phenomenon, and their skin is oedematous and itchy. During the first five years of diffuse disease (early phase), patients are weary and ill and lose weight. Arthritis, myositis, and tendon involvement are common. The fibrotic phase rapidly follows and can extend to affect most areas of skin except for the middle and lower back and buttocks. Hyperpigmentation and hypopigmentation may occur, the latter being more obvious in non-white patients. Rapid progression of skin disease is accompanied by increased risks of renal failure (often presenting as hypertensive renal crisis) and of pulmonary interstitial, early cardiac, and gastrointestinal disease.

After about five years (late phase) the constitutional symptoms usually subside. This atrophic phase may last for many years; musculoskeletal problems lead to deformity and wasting and existing visceral disease often progresses, though the risk of new organs being affected is reduced. Antibodies to scleroderma-70 (topoisomerase-1) are found in 25% of patients overall but are more characteristic of diffuse cutaneous scleroderma.

"Scleroderma sine scleroderma"

Some patients have scleroderma without their skin being affected, although they may have Raynaud's phenomenon. Patients present with complications of an internal organ such as restrictive pulmonary disease, cardiac failure, hypertensive renal crisis, or malabsorption and pseudo-obstruction. The presence of anticentromere, scleroderma-70, or antinucleolar antibodies can be helpful in making a definitive diagnosis.

Treatment

Although there is no cure for scleroderma, management tailored to the stage and subset of the disease can improve quality and length of life. Treatments include those for Raynaud's phenomenon itself, angiotensin converting enzyme inhibitors (such as captopril) for hypertension, omeprazole for oesophageal reflux, and digital sympathectomy for a critically ischaemic finger.

Raynaud's phenomenon, scleroderma, and overlap syndromes

Management of scleroderma

- Explanation and support—scleroderma is chronic and distressing for patients and their families
- Treat vascular abnormalities as for Raynaud's phenomenon
- Treat individual symptoms (such as omeprazole for oesophagitis)
- In early phase of diffuse form use immunosuppressive drugs (cyclophosphamide, methotrexate, antithymocyte globulin)
- In later stages consider antifibrotic drugs (such as penicillamine, interferon)

If the diffuse form of the disease is identified in its early oedematous stage, immunosuppressive drugs such as cyclophosphamide, methotrexate, and antithymocyte globulin are probably appropriate, followed by an antifibrotic drug such as penicillamine or interferon alfa or beta. Some of these drugs are used only in specialist centres in clinical trials, and early referral to such centres is strongly recommended. Fibrosis in the lungs, heart, and gut may develop after the skin changes stop progressing, which argues for long term use of an antifibrotic drug. The drug should not be withdrawn until the disease has been quiescent for at least a year.

The complications associated with internal organs being affected—such as cardiac arrhythmias, hypertensive renal crisis, pulmonary vascular disease, bacterial overgrowth, and oesophageal reflux—must be treated individually. Scleroderma is usually a lifelong and potentially life threatening disease. It requires accurate staging, suitable treatment, and sympathetic management, with emotional and physical support for patients and their families.

Overlap syndromes

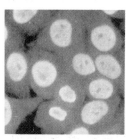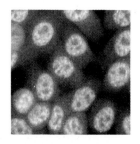
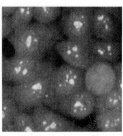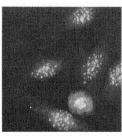

Common immunofluorescent patterns seen on testing for antinuclear antibodies: (top left) *homogeneous*—typical of antibodies to DNA, with or without histones; (top right) *speckled*—typical of antibodies to Ro, La, Sm, and RNP; (bottom left) *nucleolar*—typical of scleroderma; (bottom right) *centromere*—mainly found with limited cutaneous scleroderma.

Links between various antinuclear antibodies and autoimmune rheumatic diseases

Antibodies to Jo-1
Jo-1 antigen is a tRNA histidyl synthetase
Antibodies are present in about 30% of patients with myositis

Antibodies to scleroderma-70
Antigen is topoisomerase-1, a DNA charging enzyme
Antibodies are present in about 25% of patients with scleroderma

Antibodies to Sm, RNP, Ro, and La
Antigens are varying combinations of RNA and protein
Antibodies to Sm are present in 5–30% of patients with systemic lupus erythematosus
Antibodies to Ro and La are present in many patients with systemic lupus erythematosus or Sjögrens syndrome

Antibodies to RNA
Antibodies are not disease specific

Although well established criteria for various autoimmune rheumatic diseases have emerged and been accepted in the past 20 years, some patients cannot be fitted easily into such categories. Some patients may eventually develop a well defined disease, but in other instances — such as patients with Raynaud's phenomenon, arthralgia, and presence of antinuclear antibodies only—isolated features remain the sole manifestations during long periods of follow up. True overlap syndrome occurs when a patient clearly meets the classification criteria for two or more diseases. Thus, Sjögren's syndrome and myositis are found in 20% and 5% respectively of patients who have systemic lupus erythematosus.

Historically, classification of disease has been based on particular clinical features, which are later supported by autoantibody or biochemical markers. The only exception to this general rule was the attempt made some 20 years ago to distinguish a group of patients primarily by their high titres of antibodies to ribonucleic protein. This condition—termed mixed connective tissue disease—was thought to represent a distinct rheumatic disease, with patients having a combination of arthralgias, swollen hands, Raynaud's phenomenon, oesophagitis, and myositis but lacking cerebral, pulmonary, or renal involvement. It has since become clear that many patients have antibodies to ribonucleic protein but lack these particular clinical features. In addition, other patients have these clinical features but lack this antibody specifically, and many patients who initially seem to fit this classification eventually develop scleroderma (usually) or systemic lupus erythematosus (occasionally). For this reason the term undifferentiated autoimmune rheumatic disease (or undifferentiated connective tissue disease) is often preferred.

Treatment of patients with overlapping autoimmune rheumatic diseases is largely based on each individual's symptoms. Raynaud's phenomenon that occurs in these patients is treated no differently from severe idiopathic disease or Raynaud's phenomenon complicating other autoimmune rheumatic problems. Similarly, myositis in these patients will be treated by the conventional corticosteroids and other immunosuppressive drugs (notably azathioprine, methotrexate, or cyclophosphamide). Oesophagitis in these patients is treated in the same way as in those who have sclerodactyly or scleroderma.

The box of subsets of scleroderma is adapted from E C LeRoy *et al*, *J Rheumatol* 1988;**15**:202–5.

17 RASHES AND VASCULITIS

R A Watts, D G I Scott

Many patients with rheumatological disorders either present with a rash or develop a rash in the course of the disease. This is particularly true of the connective tissue diseases and psoriasis, which have been described elsewhere in this series. The differential diagnosis of rash and arthritis is wide, but in most cases a diagnosis can be made on the basis of history, clinical examination, and appropriate blood tests.

Infection

Several microorganisms can cause both a rash and arthritis, either by direct infection or by immune mediated mechanisms.

Streptococcal infections

Rheumatic fever is caused by an immune mediated response to group A β haemolytic streptococcal pharyngitis. It is rare in the developed world, but recent outbreaks have been reported in the United States and Europe. Most cases occur in people aged 5–16. The characteristic skin lesion is erythema marginatum. The arthritis affects large joints and migrates from joint to joint, each joint being affected for only two or three days, and lasts overall for three weeks. Nodules may develop over bony prominences; other features include chorea and carditis. Infections are treated with penicillin and anti-inflammatory drugs.

A reactive arthritis can occur after infections with group A and possibly group G streptococci. The arthritis is more prolonged, lasting for two to three months, and does not migrate between joints. It may be accompanied by a vasculitic rash.

Neisserial infections

Disseminated infection with *Neisseria gonorrhoeae* is three to five times more common in women than men. Urethritis or cervicitis is often asymptomatic. There is an initial bacteraemic phase with a migratory polyarthritis and typical skin lesions that may be maculopapular, vesicular, or pustular. Tenosynovitis of the hand, wrist, or ankle is common in established disease. *N gonorrhoeae* is the most common cause of a bacterial arthritis in adults (typically aged 15–30). The organism is usually isolated from a pustule or the genitourinary tract but can be isolated from blood or synovial fluid. It is treated with penicillin.

Infection with *N meningitidis* is associated with a widespread haemorrhagic pustular rash, particularly over the buttocks and legs, and can rapidly become life threatening. Diagnosis is confirmed by blood culture, and it is treated with penicillin. A self limiting polyarthritis may develop three to five days after the rash, which is not influenced by antibiotic treatment.

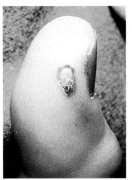
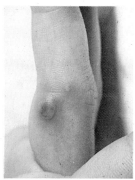

Gonococcal pustules in disseminated infection with *Neisseria gonorrhoeae.*

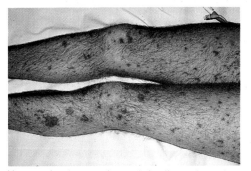

Haemorrhagic pustular rash in disseminated infection with *Neisseria meningitidis.*

Rashes and vasculitis

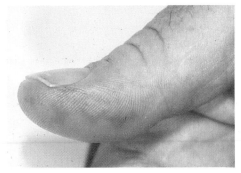

Janeway lesions in infective endocarditis.

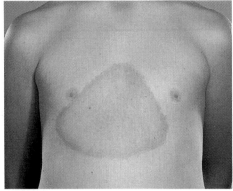

Erythema chronicum migrans at site of tick bite in Lyme disease.

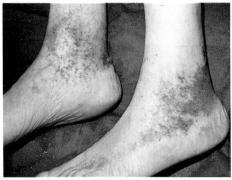

Vasculitic rash in cryoglobulinaemia.

Infective endocarditis

Several organisms—including streptococci, staphylococci, gram negative bacilli, and coxiella—can cause endocarditis. Polyarthritis may be accompanied by splinter haemorrhages, Janeway lesions (red macules on the thenar and hypothenar eminences), Osler's nodes (tender papules over the extremities of fingers and toes), and clubbing. Diagnosis is made by blood culture and echocardiography.

Lyme disease

Lyme disease is caused by the spirochaete *Borrelia burgdorferi* and is transmitted by a bite from an ixodid tick. The earliest feature is the typical rash, erythema chronicum migrans, which occurs at the site of the bite. Patients are often asymptomatic at this stage. The lesion begins as a red macule or papule that expands to form an annular erythematous lesion with an indurated centre. Secondary lesions may develop. Within a few weeks of onset a migratory polyarthritis may develop; in a few patients this becomes a chronic intermittent large joint arthropathy. Other systemic features include meningitis, encephalitis, radiculopathy, and cardiac conduction defects. Diagnosis is made by a serological test for borrelia antibodies. Early disease is treated with tetracycline, while disseminated disease should be treated with a cephalosporin or penicillin.

Rubella

Rubella virus causes a mild acute illness with a characteristic maculopapular rash and lymphadenopathy that are typically postauricular. A self limiting symmetrical polyarthritis may follow, especially in young women. Chronic joint disease does not occur.

Parvovirus

Parvovirus B19 is the cause of fifth disease or erythema infectiosum in childhood. The characteristic skin lesion is a "slapped cheek" erythema, which may be associated with a reticular rash over the trunk. An acute self limiting symmetrical polyarthritis occurs, typically in young adult women, and can last for up to one year. A rise in IgM titre is diagnostic, and autoantibodies may be present transiently.

Other infections

Hepatitis B infection can present with a small vessel vasculitis during the acute illness. Chronic hepatitis B antigenaemia may be associated with classic polyarteritis nodosa. Mixed cryoglobulinaemia may also occur after infection with hepatitis A, B, or C, and patients may present with a vasculitic rash. HIV infection is associated with an increased occurrence of Reiter's syndrome, psoriatic arthritis, and vasculitis that may affect small and medium vessels.

Drugs

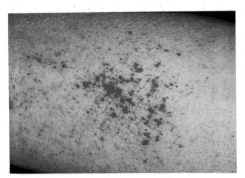

Maculopapular eruption caused by reaction to sulphasalazine (Salazopyrin).

Skin eruptions are a common complication of many drugs, including those used to treat arthritis. They are often mild but may be life threatening.

Non-steroidal anti-inflammatory drugs can be associated with mild maculopapular reactions at any stage of treatment. Phototoxicity is now rare (it was particularly associated with Opren).

Penicillamine can cause pruritus and maculopapular rashes early in treatment, while lichenoid or bullous lesions occur later. It can also induce a lupus-like illness.

Gold treatment—About 15% of patients treated with gold develop a rash, usually a non-specific maculopapular scaling eruption. Severe erythroderma is rare but can be life threatening.

Sulphasalazine—The sulphonamide part of this drug can cause a maculopapular rash and occasionally toxic epidermal necrolysis.

Immunisation with influenza or rubella vaccine or tetanus toxoid can induce a polyarthritis, which is usually transient. Chronic arthritis has been reported after immunisation, but the exact relation between the arthritis and immunisation is unclear.

Miscellaneous connective tissue disorders

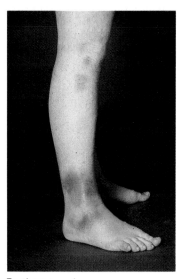

Erythema nodosum occurring in acute sarcoidosis.

Erythema nodosum

Erythema nodosum is characterised by warm tender erythematous nodules over the extensor surfaces of limbs. Individual nodules tend to resolve over three to six weeks without leaving scars. Erythema nodosum may be associated with a periarthritis, particularly of the ankles and wrists, and there are several causes of the condition. The combination of erythema nodosum, periarthritis, and bilateral hilar lymphadenopathy (seen in radiographs) is diagnostic of acute sarcoidosis and is almost always self limiting. Chronic sarcoidosis is a multisystem disease in which a destructive arthropathy and papular infiltrative skin lesions may develop. Serum concentrations of angiotensin converting enzyme are often raised in active systemic sarcoidosis.

Still's disease

This is a systemic illness with a high swinging fever, polyarthritis, and a typical evanescent skin rash. The lesions are pink macules that are most prominent during episodes of fever. Patients are seronegative for rheumatoid factor and antinuclear antibodies, and blood cultures are sterile. The condition is treated with anti-inflammatory drugs or corticosteroids. The typical age of onset is under 5, but it can occur in adults.

Acute febrile neutrophilic dermatosis (Sweet's syndrome)

This condition occurs in young women and comprises four main features: fever, painful red skin plaques, leucocytosis, and a dermal infiltrate with neutrophils. It is associated with myelodysplasia and leukaemia. It is treated with corticosteroids or other immunosuppressive agents.

Livedo reticularis

Livedo reticularis is characterised by persistent patchy reddish-blue mottling of the legs (and occasionally arms) which is exacerbated by cold weather. It may lead to ulceration and is associated with vascular thrombosis (Sneddon's syndrome) and the presence of antiphospholipid antibodies.

Vasculitis

The vasculitides are a heterogeneous group of uncommon diseases characterised by inflammatory cell infiltration and necrosis of blood vessel walls. Systemic vasculitis can rapidly become life threatening, so early accurate diagnosis and treatment is vital. Vasculitis may be primary (such as polyarteritis nodosa) or secondary to connective tissue disease (such as rheumatoid arthritis), infection, or malignancy. The severity of vasculitis is related to the size and site of the vessels affected. Classification is also based on vessel size, which reflects treatment strategies.

Rashes and vasculitis

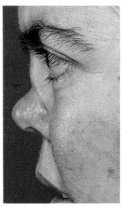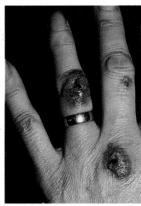

Wegener's granulomatosis: (left) typical saddle nose deformity (reproduced with patient's permission); (right) vasculitic rash.

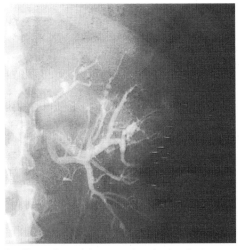

Coeliac axis arteriogram showing typical aneurysm in polyarteritis nodosa.

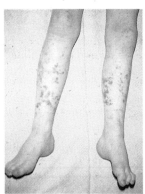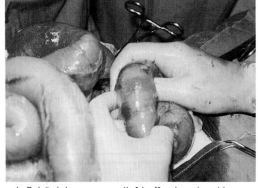

Small vessel vasculitis in Henoch-Schönlein purpura: (left) affecting the skin; (right) affecting the gut.

Systemic necrotising arteritis

This group of conditions includes the major necrotising vasculitides: classic polyarteritis nodosa, microscopic polyangiitis (also called microscopic polyarteritis nodosa), Wegener's granulomatosis, and Churg-Strauss syndrome, with necrosis of medium and small arteries. They may occur at any age and are not uncommon in elderly people. Primary systemic vasculitis is slightly more common in men. The annual incidence is about 30 cases per million people. The symptoms of vasculitis depends on the size and site of vessel affected and on the individual condition.

Wegener's granulomatosis is characterised by a granulomatous vasculitis of the upper and lower respiratory tracts and glomerulonephritis, but almost any organ system can be affected. The lungs are affected in 45% of patients at diagnosis. Symptoms of the ear, nose, and throat (such as epistaxis, crusting, and deafness) are particularly associated with this condition and should be sought in all patients with suspected vasculitis. Patients with limited Wegener's granulomatosis—disease without renal impairment—may have a better prognosis. Biopsy of affected organs shows a necrotising arteritis, often with formation of granulomas. Microscopic polyangiitis is a vasculitis of medium arteries and small vessels and mainly affects the kidneys.

Churg-Strauss syndrome is characterised by atopy (in particular late onset asthma), pulmonary involvement (75% of patients have radiographic evidence of infiltration), and eosinophilia. These features can develop several years before the start of systemic disease. Cardiac involvement is a particular feature of Churg-Strauss syndrome and is a determinant of prognosis.

Polyarteritis nodosa is a multisystem vasculitis characterised by formation of aneurysms in medium sized arteries. Patients present with a constitutional illness, often associated with a rash, mononeuritis multiplex, or vascular hypertension. Polyarteritis nodosa may be confined to the skin. Angiography shows the presence of typical aneurysms. Classic polyarteritis nodosa has been associated with chronic hepatitis B antigenaemia, especially in the United States, but this is rare in the United Kingdom.

Kawasaki disease (mucocutaneous lymph node syndrome) is an acute vasculitis that primarily affects infants and young children. It presents as fever, rash, lymphadenopathy, and palmoplantar erythema. Coronary arteries become affected in up to a quarter of untreated patients, and this can lead to myocardial ischaemia and infarction.

Small vessel vasculitis

Small vessel vasculitis (leucocytoclastic or hypersensitivity vasculitis) is usually confined to the skin but may be part of a systemic illness. The rash is purpuric and sometimes palpable and occurs in dependent areas. The lesions may become bullous and ulcerate. Nailfold infarcts occur. Biopsies show a cellular infiltrate of small vessels often with leucocytoclasis (fragmented polymorphonuclear cells and nuclear dust). There are several causes of small vessel vasculitis, drugs and infection being the most common.

Henoch-Schönlein purpura is a form of small vessel vasculitis that occurs mainly in children and young adults. Patients present with rash, arthritis, abdominal pain, and sometimes renal impairment. Deposits of IgA can be detected in the skin and renal mesangium.

Large vessel vasculitis

This group of diseases includes giant cell arteritis and Takayasu's arteritis. The second condition is uncommon and affects young adults, who present with a non-specific illness and later with loss of pulses and claudication, especially of the upper limbs.

Investigation of vasculitis

Assessing inflammation
- Urine analysis (proteinuria, haematuria, casts)
- Renal function tests (creatinine clearance, 24 hour protein excretion)
- Blood count (total, white blood cells, eosinophils)
- Acute phase response (erythrocyte sedimentation rate, C reactive protein)
- Liver function tests

Immunological tests
- Autoantibodies (rheumatoid factor, antinuclear antibodies, antineutrophil cytoplasmic antibodies, anticardiolipin antibodies)
- Complement and immune complexes
- Cryoglobulins

Differential diagnosis
- Blood cultures
- Viral serology (hepatitis B, cytomegalovirus)
- Echocardiography

Specific investigations
- Radiographs of chest and sinus
- Biopsy of affected organs (especially kidney)
- Angiography

Important mimics of vasculitis

- Subacute bacterial endocarditis
- Atrial myxoma
- Cholesterol embolism
- Antiphospholipid antibody syndrome

Aims of management of vasculitis

- Induction of remission
- Maintenance of remission
- Recognition and early treatment of relapse
- Avoidance of drug toxicity

Treatment regimens for cyclophosphamide

Continuous low oral dose
Cyclophosphamide	2 mg/kg/day
Prednisolone	1 mg/kg/day

Oral pulse
Cyclophosphamide	5 mg/kg/day × 3 days
Prednisolone	100 mg/day × 3 days

Intravenous pulse*
Cyclophosphamide	10–15 mg/kg†
Prednisolone	1 g

*Pulse frequency: fortnightly (×6), every three weeks (×2), monthly (×6). Adjusted according to clinical response and toxicity.

†Dose adjusted according to white cell count, renal function, and clinical response. White cell count should be checked 7, 10, and 14 days after the first two pulses and immediately before subsequent pulses.

Investigation of vasculitis

Investigation is directed towards establishing the diagnosis, the organs affected, and disease activity.

Urine analysis is the most important investigation since prognosis is determined mainly by the extend of renal impairment. Detection of proteinuria or haematuria in a patient with systemic illness requires immediate further investigation and is a medical emergency.

Blood tests—Leucocytosis suggests either primary vasculitis or infection, while leucopenia is associated with vasculitis secondary to a connective tissue disease. Eosinophilia suggests Churg-Strauss syndrome or a drug reaction.

Liver function tests—Abnormal results suggest either viral infection (hepatitis A, B, or C) or may be non-specific.

Immunology—Rheumatoid factors and antinuclear antibodies may indicate vasculitis associated with connective tissue disease. Measurement of antineutrophil cytoplasmic antibodies by indirect immunofluorescence is now widely available: cytoplasmic antineutrophil cytoplasmic antibodies are strongly associated with Wegener's granulomatosis, while perinuclear antineutrophil cytoplasmic antibodies are less so. Complement concentrations are low in infection and systemic lupus erythematosus but high in primary vasculitis.

Other investigations—Aneurysms can be revealed by angiography. Blood cultures, viral serology, and echocardiography are important to exclude infection and other conditions that may present as systemic multisystem disease and hence mimic vasculitis.

Treatment and prognosis

Treatment depends on the size of vessel affected. Small vessel vasculitis without necrotising features has an excellent prognosis and can usually be treated conservatively; patients with systemic disease respond well to a short course (<3 months) of treatment with corticosteroids (20–60 mg oral prednisolone). Large vessel vasculitis also has a good prognosis and responds well to corticosteroids (40–60 mg oral prednisolone), but treatment is usually needed for more than a year. The dose of corticosteroid should be rapidly reduced according to clinical and laboratory parameters, with the aim of reducing the dose to 10 mg or less within six months.

The introduction of cyclophosphamide has dramatically improved the prognosis of systemic necrotising vasculitis. Cyclophosphamide can be given either as continuous low dose oral treatment or as intermittent pulse therapy. The second method is preferred because of lower toxicity with intravenous therapy: cyclophosphamide's main toxic effects are haemorrhagic cystitis and formation of bladder tumours, and pulse therapy is significantly less toxic to the bladder than continuous oral therapy. Mesna may reduce this toxicity. Fertile men should be offered sperm storage before they are given treatment; ovarian function is less severely affected with pulse regimens.

Treatment with cyclophosphamide is continued for at least six months after remission before it is replaced by oral treatment with azathioprine. Survival has improved, but many patients require prolonged treatment (5–10 years) and there is still a substantial relapse rate, as high as 50% with continuous oral cyclophosphamide.

Plasmapheresis is reserved for patients with pulmonary haemorrhage and severe renal disease. Intravenous treatment with immunoglobulin is effective for Kawasaki disease, but its role in other vasculitides is uncertain at present. Co-trimoxazole may be used for limited Wegener's granulomatosis. Weekly treatment with oral methotrexate is a possible alternative to azathioprine.

The photograph of erythema migrans due to Lyme disease was reproduced with permission of Dr J E White, University of Southampton.

18 LABORATORY TESTS

Charles Mackworth-Young, David A Isenberg

Haematological investigations

A full blood count and erythrocyte sedimentation rate are used to monitor disease activity, to assess the effects of drug treatment, to exclude factors such as dietary deficiency or haemolysis that may be contributing to the morbidity of a rheumatological disease, and (rarely) to exclude a primary haematological malignancy that can mimic various forms of arthritis. The erythrocyte sedimentation rate is considered in detail in the section on acute phase proteins.

Anaemia of chronic disease

Inflammatory arthritides are associated with normochromic normocytic anaemia. The pathogenesis is multifactorial and probably involves various cytokines, particularly interleukin 1. Major factors contributing to such anaemia include reduced iron supplies (impaired absorption and transportation and failure to release iron stores), reduced concentrations of erythropoietin, ineffective erythropoiesis, and abnormal development of erythroid progenitor cells. Moderate anaemia may reflect disease activity, but a haemoglobin concentration below 100 g/l usually has another cause.

Iron deficiency anaemia

Hypochromic microcytic anaemia with a low serum iron concentration and raised total iron binding capacity may be due to components of the rheumatological disease itself—such as the oesophagitis present in some patients with scleroderma—or to dietary insufficiency of iron, but it is often a complication of treatment with non-steroidal anti-inflammatory drugs. Apart from causing upper gastrointestinal tract ulcers, these drugs may affect platelet function, enhancing the tendency to chronic low grade blood loss.

Megaloblastic anaemia

In most cases macrocytosis reflects folate deficiency, but pernicious anaemia is associated with some of the autoimmune rheumatic diseases, notably rheumatoid arthritis. Macrocytosis is a recognised complication of methotrexate (a folate antagonist) and azathioprine, drugs now widely prescribed in patients with rheumatoid and psoriatic arthritis.

Haemolytic anaemia

Autoimmune haemolytic anaemia occurs in up to 10% of patients with systemic lupus erythematosus and may rarely occur in association with rheumatoid arthritis and other autoimmune rheumatic diseases.

Platelet abnormalities

Platelet abnormalities are often seen in rheumatic disorders, the most common being a mild to moderate thrombocytosis. In rheumatoid arthritis thrombocytopenia may occur as a side effect of gold or penicillamine treatment. An autoimmune thrombocytopenia (usually chronic but occasionally acute) occurs in up to 20% of patients with lupus and in patients with the primary antiphospholipid antibody syndrome. In some of these patients it has been possible to demonstrate the presence of antiplatelet antibodies. Rarely, an idiopathic thrombocytopenia precedes the development of lupus.

White blood cell abnormalities

Felty's syndrome — the association of rheumatoid arthritis with leucopenia (predominantly neutropenia) and splenomegaly (and often leg ulcers)—is rare. Leucopenia, particularly lymphopenia, is common in lupus. Bone marrow suppression is a well recognised complication of immunosuppressive drugs such as azathioprine, methotrexate, and cyclophosphamide that are used to treat severe rheumatoid arthritis, psoriatic arthritis, and lupus.

Leukocytosis is occasionally found in flares of lupus. Less common abnormalities, such as monocytopenia and eosinophilia in rheumatoid arthritis and basopenia in lupus, are well described.

Coagulation abnormalities

Lupus anticoagulant is discussed in the section about antiphospholipid antibodies.

Biochemical investigations

Acute phase response

This response defines a coordinated set of systemic and local events associated with the inflammation that is the consequence of tissue damage. The term is misleading in that the changes may occur in both acute and chronic inflammation. About 30 acute phase proteins are known. Elevated serum concentrations of these proteins often last for several days after the initiating event, and their synthesis in the liver is triggered by several cytokines—particularly interleukin 1, interleukin 6, and tumour necrosis factor. These cytokines derive from macrophages that have been activated at the site of the injury, though other cell types, such as fibroblasts and endothelial cells, are also sources. There is some specificity in these interactions: for example, the synthesis of C reactive protein is dependent on interleukin 6 whereas haptoglobin is influenced by all three of the cytokines mentioned above.

It is impractical and unnecessary to measure all aspects of the acute phase response, and the most widely used measurements are probably erythrocyte sedimentation rate, C reactive protein, and plasma viscosity. Less common measurements are serum amyloid A protein, haptoglobin, and fibrinogen.

Erythrocyte sedimentation rate (the sedimentation of erythrocytes in 1 hour at 1 g) depends on the degree of aggregation of these cells and the packed cell volume. The process of aggregation is affected by plasma proteins including fibrinogen, α_2 macroglobulin, and immunoglobulins. The sedimentation rate thus reflects alterations in a variety of proteins. Technical modifications, such as "seditainer tubes," have reduced costs and the risk of infection from contaminated blood.

Plasma viscosity differs from the erythrocyte sedimentation rate in that it is not affected by red cells, is easier to standardise, and is independent of sex. It offers several advantages over the erythrocyte sedimentation rate but is greatly dependent on the concentration of fibrinogen. Both tests are widely available, simple to establish, relatively inexpensive, and are used as general screens for many diseases. They also reflect disease activity in patients with inflammatory rheumatic disease (such as rheumatoid arthritis, psoriatic arthritis, and lupus).

C reactive protein—The serum concentrations of this protein fluctuate more rapidly than the erythrocyte sedimentation rate or plasma viscosity but may not rise in the presence of relatively mild inflammation. Patients with active lupus invariably have raised erythrocyte sedimentation rates, whereas the C reactive protein is normal or only slightly raised unless a patient has synovitis, respiratory disease, or a concomitant infection. Indeed, the concentration of C reactive protein is often used to distinguish infection from disease activity in lupus patients. The protein's short half life offers the opportunity to monitor the response of an infection to antibiotic treatment.

Liver function

Abnormalities in liver function may reflect disease activity in some rheumatic diseases (for example, alkaline phosphatase activity in rheumatoid arthritis and liver enzyme tests in polymyositis). Raised enzyme activities may also be due to damage from drugs used to treat rheumatic diseases. Many of the drugs used to treat rheumatic diseases—notably methotrexate, azathioprine, cyclophosphamide, and sulphasalazine—may damage the liver. The recommended frequency of hepatic monitoring varies, but baseline assessment is advisable before starting any of the drugs mentioned above.

Many of the enzymes and proteins measured do not originate solely from the liver. Thus a common cause of an isolated rise in alkaline phosphatase activity is Paget's disease, in which the patient's bone is the real site of origin. However, elevated alkaline phosphatase activity has been recorded in patients with temporal arteritis, polymyalgia rheumatica, scleroderma, and, occasionally, systemic lupus erythematosus.

Renal function

Abnormal renal function may also be a component of a rheumatic disease (such as after deposition of uric acid crystals in the kidneys of patients with gout) or a consequence of treatment. Measurement of plasma creatinine concentration is widely used as a test of renal dysfunction. However, it is not sensitive: the creatinine clearance must fall below 30 ml/min (about a third of normal values) before the plasma creatinine concentration becomes abnormally high.

Twenty four hour urine collections depend on the reliability of the patient. Serial estimations of urine protein concentration do help to gauge the response to treatment in, for example, patients with lupus or with amyloidosis complicating rheumatoid arthritis (an accurate measure of creatinine clearance, the chromium-51 labelled EDTA test, is a widely available and useful assessment of glomerular function).

Plasma urea concentration is a less sensitive measure than the plasma creatinine concentration and is influenced by several factors, including rate of protein metabolism and fluid balance. Other measures exist, including the detection of certain enzymes such as the lyzosymal enzyme N-acetyl-D-glucosaminidase, and proximal tubule function can be useful in certain circumstances.

Bone calcium

The main diseases of bone that are presented to rheumatologists are osteoporosis, osteomalacia, and Paget's disease. Thus, the most commonly measured markers are the serum alkaline phosphatase activity and serum calcium concentration. Both tend to be normal in osteoporosis, while a raised alkaline phosphatase activity of bone origin is the key feature of Paget's disease. Severe cases of osteomalacia are associated with hypocalcaemia and increased alkaline phosphatase activity. Biochemical markers for bone and cartilage turnover are being investigated but are not yet available for routine clinical tests.

Other biochemical tests

Plasma urate has been discussed earlier in the chapter about gout and hyperuricaemia. Muscle diseases and polymyositis in particular are associated with a rise in the creatine kinase activity. This enzyme occurs as three isoenzymes: creatine kinase MM originates principally from the skeletal muscle, creatine kinase BB is principally from the brain and thyroid, and creatine kinase MB arises from the myocardium and skeletal muscle. Serial measurements of creatine kinase activity often reflect disease activity in myositis, but interpretation of readings should take into account possible racial variations and the fact that vigorous exercise can dramatically but temporarily raise enzyme activity.

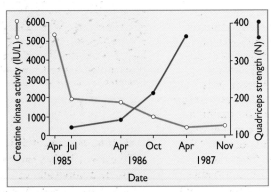

Concentration of creatine kinase falls as muscle strength improves in a patient with myositis.

Immunological investigations

Autoantibodies

Autoantibodies are immunoglobulins which bind to self antigens (molecules present in the patient's own tissues). Low concentrations of autoantibodies are present in the plasma of normal individuals, but in autoimmune conditions some of these antibodies are overexpressed. This may be due to various factors, including environmental triggers such as infection together with the genetic susceptibility of a patient. Autoantibodies may be divided into those that are directed against certain organ specific antigens (such as the acetyl choline receptor in myasthenia gravis and intrinsic factor in pernicious anaemia) and those that bind to more widespread antigens such as DNA or cardiolipin.

Raised concentrations of certain organ specific antibodies are sometimes seen in patients with rheumatic diseases (and in their relatives), which may reflect an overall increased tendency to autoimmunity in such individuals. However, autoantibodies that are not organ specific are characteristic of these conditions. Detection of autoantibodies in rheumatic disorders is generally more useful for diagnosis than for monitoring disease activity.

Rheumatoid factors

These antibodies are immunoglobulins that bind to the Fc (constant region) of IgG. Several tests are available. The classic Rose-Waaler test relies on the ability of rheumatoid factors to agglutinate sheep erythrocytes coated with antisheep immunoglobulin. Its descendant, the sheep cell agglutination test, and other tests such as the rheumatoid arthritis particle agglutination assay can be semiquantitative. Normal ranges vary between laboratories, but titres greater than 1:80 are generally considered to be positive results. These tests identify only the IgM isotype. Detection of IgG and IgA rheumatoid factors by enzyme linked immunosorbent assay (ELISA) is becoming more widely available.

A raised titre of IgM rheumatoid factor has a definite but limited value as a diagnostic test for rheumatoid arthritis. The test is positive in about 70% of patients with rheumatoid arthritis and in some patients with other disorders, including other arthritic conditions (such as lupus and Sjögren's syndrome). But in the right clinical context the test can be very useful. Oligoarticular rheumatoid arthritis may be associated with a negative test for IgM rheumatoid factor but a positive test for IgG rheumatoid factor. The clinical specificity of IgA rheumatoid factor is not clear.

Antinuclear antibodies

These are immunoglobulins that bind to antigens in the cell nucleus. These antibodies are usually detected by immunofluorescence, using murine liver or kidney cells. As with rheumatoid factor, a titre of greater than 1:80 is usually considered positive, although there is considerable variation between laboratories. A positive test for antinuclear antibodies is not diagnostic of systemic lupus erythematosus as it may occur in several conditions. In infectious diseases the test tends to be positive only transiently, and in the right clinical context a positive test is strongly suggestive of an autoimmune rheumatic disease.

With cell cultures that have a high proportion of dividing cells, antibodies to the centromere (the central portion of each chromosome) may be found; such antibodies are commonly seen in the CREST syndrome, a relatively restricted form of scleroderma.

It is often possible to characterise an antinuclear antibody more precisely, and this should be attempted for any patient with a rheumatic disorder and a positive test for antinuclear antibody.

Antibodies to DNA

Anti-DNA antibodies are usually detected by the Farr assay (a precipitation test) or by ELISA. Other tests, particularly the immunofluorescence test with *Crithidia luciliae*, are also available. *Crithidia* contains double stranded DNA, and the test is rarely positive in patients who have anything other than lupus. Although antibodies to single stranded DNA are often present in sera positive for antinuclear antibodies, detection of antibodies to double stranded DNA is diagnostically more useful for lupus. Such antibodies are often found in high titre in lupus and are especially likely to be found in patients with renal disease. They often, but unreliably, reflect disease activity, and a rise in titre may predict a flare.

The pattern of immunofluorescence varies according to which nuclear or cytoplasmic antigens are recognised. Thus homogeneous staining across the nucleus is commonly seen in lupus and reflects binding to DNA or histones. A speckled pattern of staining is characteristic of antibodies found in overlap or mixed diseases and may be due to binding to ribonucleic acid, Sm, Ro, or La proteins. Sm, Ro, and La are varying combinations of RNA and proteins (the names derive from the surnames of the patients in whom antibodies to the combinations were first found; thus Sm stands for Smith). Staining that is restricted to the nucleolus is typically seen in scleroderma.

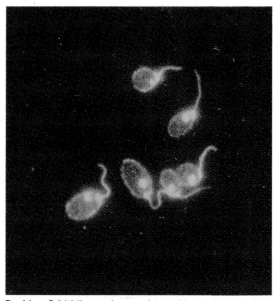

Positive *Crithidia* test in a patient with systemic lupus erythematosus.

Antibodies to extractable nuclear antigens

These antibodies can be detected by counterimmunoelectrophoresis, in which serum is tested against a saline extract of mammalian nuclei and compared with reference sera. More specific tests for each antigen (which consist of varying combinations of RNA and protein) are now available in many laboratories and are generally solid phase immunoassays.

The identification of antibodies to one or more antigen in a patient's serum can be helpful in the diagnosis of an autoimmune disease. For instance, antibodies to Sm are almost restricted to lupus (particularly in the black population). Similarly, antibodies to Ro and La (also known as SS-A and SS-B) are often found in Sjögren's syndrome. There is, however, considerable overlap between expression of clinical disease and expression of particular antibodies.

Antiphospholipid antibodies

In the rheumatological context antiphospholipid antibodies bind chiefly to negatively charged phospholipids such as cardiolipin. There are three tests available. The Venereal Disease Research Laboratory test (used in the diagnosis of syphilis) detects a proportion of such antibodies, but is of limited diagnostic value. More sensitive is the lupus anticoagulant test, which is a coagulation assay based on the partial thromboplastin time. The simplest and cheapest is the ELISA for anticardiolipin antibodies. These three tests detect slightly different but overlapping populations of antibodies.

Raised concentrations of antiphospholipid antibodies are associated with several clinical features including thrombosis (both arterial and venous), recurrent fetal loss, thrombocytopenia, and various neurological disorders. This antiphospholipid syndrome may occur in isolation or in the context of a connective tissue disease such as lupus. There is some evidence that these antibodies may directly interfere with coagulation mechanisms.

Antineutrophil cytoplasmic antibodies

These are antibodies that bind to antigens in the cytoplasm of neutrophils. The standard test is immunofluorescence on cultured neutrophils. Usually one of two patterns is seen: a diffuse "cytoplasmic" staining (cANCA) or a "peripheral" staining pattern around the edge of the cell (pANCA). cANCA and pANCA bind to several proteins, the most common being serine proteinase III and myeloperoxidase respectively. Solid phase immunoassays may be used to determine the specificity in each case.

Antibodies to proteinase III are found in about 80% of patients with Wegener's granulomatosis. Those against myeloperoxidase are common in polyarteritis nodosa but have also be identified in patients with vasculitis complicating lupus and rheumatoid arthritis. Antibodies with other specificities have been described in non-vasculitic diseases but are of limited importance.

Immunoglobulins

A general polyclonal rise in total immunoglobulin concentrations is commonly seen in many inflammatory rheumatic diseases as a non-specific reflection of an acute phase response. In Sjögren's syndrome total IgG concentrations may be substantially raised, often up to 30 g/l or more. Low concentrations of total IgA are sometimes seen in lupus, and high concentrations may be found in patients with active ankylosing spondylitis. Occasionally, patients with a primary immunodeficiency (low concentrations of one or more immunoglobulin class or subclass) may present with rheumatic disorders such as rheumatoid arthritis or lupus.

Complement

Proteins of the complement cascade play a central role in cell lysis, opsonisation of bacteria, and clearance of immune complexes. C3 and C4 components are most commonly measured (and in some laboratories CH_{50}, which is a measure of overall activity of the whole complement pathway) and are useful in screening for complement deficiencies.

As part of the acute phase response, complement proteins often show a modest rise in many inflammatory rheumatic diseases (such as rheumatoid arthritis and seronegative arthropathies). Concentrations occasionally fall if an associated vasculitis develops and so can be a useful diagnostic pointer in this situation. In diseases characterised by excess production of immune complexes (such as lupus) consumption of individual complement components may exceed production, and overall concentrations may fall. Low concentrations are usually found in active lupus and, especially in the case of renal lupus, often parallel disease activity. Thus repeated measurement may be useful for monitoring progress. Some patients, however, retain low complement concentrations when in clinical remission.

Deficiency of a complement component may occasionally be hereditary and associated with the development of lupus. Such cases are very rare, and low complement concentrations in patients with lupus are almost always acquired.

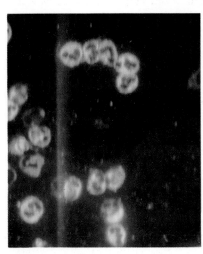
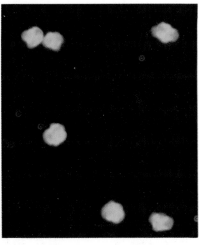

Tests for antineutrophil cytoplasmic antibodies: Positive cANCA in a patient with Wegener's granulomatosis (left); positive pANCA in a patient with polyarteritis nodosa (right).

19 THE TEAM APPROACH IN A RHEUMATOLOGY DEPARTMENT

H A Bird, Jackie Hill, Patricia le Gallez

The wide diversity of the rheumatic diseases and the many parts of the body they can affect require a multidisciplinary team in hospital, and even general practice, for managing these conditions. This article focuses on medical aspects, but surgery should not be forgotten, particularly when medical efforts fail to help.

Clinical assessments

For inflammatory polyarthritis, clinical assessment should be made in conjunction with laboratory assessments of disease activity. For some conditions, particularly soft tissue rheumatism, only clinical assessments are available and are often undertaken by nurses, physiotherapists, and occupational therapists. A daily pain score and weekly articular index, performed by a nurse, can complement daily measurements of temperature, pulse, and blood pressure in hospital patients. Physiotherapists may target their assessment to a single worst affected joint. Occupational therapists focus on functional assessment, possibly with the hospital activity questionnaire. Radiological assessment is also a crucial measure of outcome and should not be ignored.

Various scales are available to allow patients to depict their pain and stiffness. These may be incorporated in a daily diary card for use when a patient returns home. The Ritchie articular pain index should be performed by a therapist. Measuring grip strength with a sphygmomanometer bag is a more composite assessment of muscle power and joint integrity in the hand as well as joint inflammation. Clinical and laboratory assessment may be combined into a single cumulative index (such as the Lansbury or Mallya-Mace). Alternatively, use of separate assessments may convey more precise information about the effects of different treatments.

Monitoring drug toxicity

Even simple analgesic and non-steroidal anti-inflammatory drugs have side effects, and more potent compounds such as gold and immunosuppressive drugs have more severe potential side effects. Some drugs require hospital monitoring; for others, shared care with a patient's general practitioner may be feasible. Optimum care is a balance between improvement and the least risk of toxicity.

Patients must be fully educated to ensure compliance with drug regimens and to reduce morbidity from toxicity. Pharmacists can help in preparing patient information sheets. Routine monitoring can be safely delegated to a nurse trained to detect toxic side effects and to record relevant variables, such as platelet count, as well as to give injections. Pharmacists should also advise on compliance and packaging: many patients with arthritic hands find it hard to open blister packs and child proof containers.

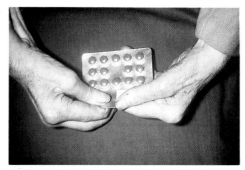

Patients with arthritic hands have difficulty opening blister packs.

Roles of team members

Physiotherapists

Many patients with arthritis would benefit from an early physiotherapy assessment and subsequent follow up. Treatment should be at the physiotherapist's discretion. Patients should be taught a self help programme as well as receiving hospital outpatient treatment as required since many arthritides are characterised by periods of remission alternating with flares.

Various forms of electrotherapy are available such as infra red radiation, pulsed short wave diathermy, ultrasound, and microwave therapy. Wax and oil baths may be used for the hands and feet, while hydrocollator packs or icepacks may be more appropriate for larger joints. Many patients, particularly those with large joint arthritis, benefit from hydrotherapy.

Some of these treatments can be improvised at home. Exercises in the local swimming baths can replace hydrotherapy to a limited extent; a hot water bottle, electric pad, or hot towel can mimic a wax or oil bath; and a large packet of frozen peas, wrapped in a teatowel, mimics an icepack around the offending joint.

Team approach in a rheumatology department

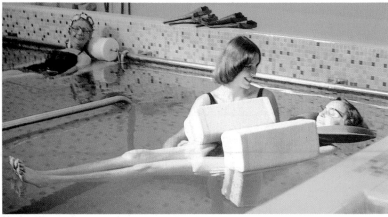

Hydrotherapy.

An acutely inflamed joint should be rested but still put through a passive range of movement. Otherwise active physiotherapy is to be encouraged, except possibly in certain types of fibromyalgia, when electrotherapy and rest may be more effective. A common criticism of physical treatments is the lack of evidence of benefit on outcome from controlled trials. It should, however, be remembered that symptomatic relief is an end in itself, that placebo responses are themselves worthwhile, and that multiple methods of treatment are appropriate for conditions comprising a mixture of active inflammation and established functional disability.

Occupational therapists

Patients, particularly those with severe arthritis, should be offered early occupational therapy assessment and subsequent follow up. This should concentrate initially on the provision of aids to improve independence, and later should focus on aspects of rehabilitation if deformity has not been controlled by medical and surgical means.

An occupational therapy department should contain a kitchen, bedroom, bathroom, and toilet. Various aids can be provided as required. When domestic adaptations are required (such as provision of a stairlift or replacement of a bath with a shower) liaison will be with the social services or housing department of the local council and sometimes with a medical social worker.

Aids to mobility may provide partial weight relief (sticks, crutches, and walking frames) or complete weight relief (patient propelled wheelchair, attendant propelled wheelchair, powered wheelchair, and outdoor vehicles) are available. These may be provided by an occupational therapist or a physiotherapist according to local custom. Although patients' work and self esteem remain paramount, hobbies should not be forgotten. Arthritic change often occurs slowly, allowing the learning of new techniques. Typing, needlework, sport, and playing musical instruments need not be discounted, though sometimes specialist collaboration with trainers or teachers may be required to ensure that patients achieve optimal performance in spite of their diseased joints.

Nurses

All rheumatology inpatients are likely to be allocated a personal "named" nurse, who will implement the nursing process and plan appropriate nursing care. It will often make sense for the nurse to supervise the provision of resting splints (ensuring that joints at rest are in their position of maximum function) in collaboration with a physiotherapist or occupational therapist. The help of orthotists or appliance makers is also often required.

The ward nurse may have the best chance to provide education to inpatients, while a clinic run by a nurse practitioner may be established to provide education, information, and counselling for outpatients. However, in some departments education remains the province of the physiotherapist or occupational therapist. Detailed education from each is often most helpful to patients, reflecting the differences between each specialty's training.

Appliance makers

Deformed feet need special shoes, and chiropodists (podiatrists) should work in collaboration with orthotists to provide this. If deformity in the feet is not corrected early, secondary strain is placed on other joints in the lower limb. Problems in the legs are often accentuated by a patient being overweight, and the help of a dietician may be required.

Calipers may be required if deformity is severe, particularly if surgery is not indicated on medical grounds. For milder sorts of arthritis lightweight splints are helpful (for example, "futura" wrist splints). Many patients use plasterzote rest splints in the hope of preventing deformity at night; these are alternated with flexible lightweight supports (or even elasticated bandages) for daytime activity.

In some types of inflammatory arthritis the contour of joints changes relatively quickly. Using a succession of inexpensive temporary and adaptable appliances, obtained at regular visits to an appliance maker, may be more beneficial than ordering a custom built rigid appliance such as shoes that remain inflexible as the foot contour changes.

Medical social workers

Disabled arthritic patients are likely to qualify for various grants and concessions. Information about these is traditionally provided by medical social workers, who are often no longer based in hospitals. In some departments nurses or other therapists have taken on this role. The local authority social worker will, however, be able to advise on the possibilities for rehousing and, in conjunction with the disablement resettlement officer, on changes of career if these become appropriate. Occasionally, industrial occupational retraining may be necessary.

Rheumatologists

Hospital based rheumatologists traditionally act as coordinators for the team approach. They are the only team member adequately trained to make a diagnosis, estimate the prognosis, and then balance the possible hazards of treatment against their likely benefits.

In cases of systemic polyarthritis, physicians should be on guard for damage to organs other than the joints that may complicate the clinical picture. Patient education requires supervision, and physicians remain the only member of the team qualified to prescribe the full panoply of drugs. Sometimes the need for systemic drugs may be averted by the use of local intraarticular injections, which are traditionally given by physicians. Physicians are also best placed to integrate the various efforts of other health workers, with knowledge of prognosis.

Surgeons

Combined medical and surgical clinics for treating rheumatoid diseases are valuable for training purposes, but space does not permit a description of surgical techniques here.

Organisational arrangements are important since surgeons and their deputies may be called away to provide emergency cover. Orthopaedic surgeons often specialise in treating certain joints. It is debatable whether patients who require multijoint surgery are best admitted to a rheumatology bed, transferring to the care of each orthopaedic surgeon in turn, or whether such patients can be managed from orthopaedic wards, and the decision depends on local circumstances. Certainly the importance of rheumatologists in rehabilitation should not be forgotten. In addition, patients are often elderly and require a thorough medical examination before surgery.

Community or hospital management?

There has been a trend for outpatient facilities to become more important in the treatment of arthritic patients, as retention of the patients' mobility, rather than enforced bed rest, has become preferred. In turn there has been a tendency for some hospital facilities to be moved into the community, particularly when large health centres have access to their own physiotherapists, occupational therapists, and nurse practitioners.

For some aspects of management, however, the superior facilities in hospital will remain essential. The Primary Care Rheumatological Society has done much to foster interest in the specialty in general practice and the community, thereby relieving some of the strain on hard pressed hospitals, but it is unlikely that this approach will completely obviate the need for the more comprehensive facilities enjoyed by hospital physicians.

Indeed, the wide diversity of specialists now needed to adequately remedy all types of arthritis is likely only to be found in the hospital. The way forward is probably regular intermittent hospital review, ensuring all patients have continued access to the most recent developments, with intermediate care being provided by local general practices.

Many hospitals are taking the initiative in supervising community care for medical specialties, and it remains to be seen to what extent the advent of hospital trusts and fundholding general practices will influence the pattern that is evolving. Certainly, continued collaboration between hospital and community services remains essential for home visits, which might be recommended towards the end of a patient's hospital stay, when the occupational therapist—sometimes accompanied by the physiotherapist, nursing sister, or medical social worker—ensures that the patient is not a risk to themselves when discharged.

Supporting organisations

Several patient self help groups have sprung up in the past decade. Many patients find it helpful to meet people with similar problems. Others have argued that these groups sometimes attract the worst afflicted patients, so that attending group meetings alarms rather than reassures. If physicians ensure that relevant and accurate information is provided patients are able to decide for themselves.

Rheumatologists are aided substantially by two national charities.

Arthritis Care concentrates on improving facilities for patients with arthritis. A telephone helpline (0800 289 170) is provided between 12 pm and 4 pm on Mondays to Fridays, and some patient information leaflets and a regular newspaper are also produced. The organisation runs hotels where disabled arthritic patients can have a holiday. More information is available from Arthritis Care, 18 Stephenson Way, London NW1 2HD (telephone 0171 916 1500).

The Arthritis and Rheumatism Council has a primary role in supporting research into the cause and treatment of arthritis, though a proportion of its funds are set aside for educating patients (as well as students and doctors). The council produces an excellent series of booklets and pamphlets which give details and answer common questions about specific diseases. A full list of leaflets available, which are free of charge apart from postage, can be obtained from the Arthritis and Rheumatism Council, Copeman House, St Mary's Court, St Mary's Gate, Chesterfield, Derbyshire S41 7TD (telephone 01246 558033).

20 EPIDEMIOLOGY OF RHEUMATIC DISEASES

T D Spector

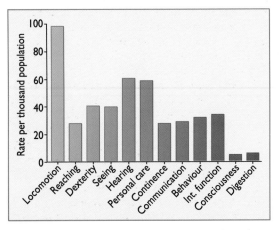

Prevalence of types of disability in Great Britain
(OPCS survey)

In developed countries musculoskeletal diseases are the commonest causes of disability in adults and, including back pain, of time lost from work. The commonest single cause of disability is osteoarthritis, which can affect the knee, spine, or hip. Osteoporosis leading to fractures is probably the second greatest public health problem, with more than one in three women likely to sustain an osteoporotic fracture at the wrist, hip, or spine during their lifetime.

Rheumatoid arthritis accounts for up to 50% of the workload of most rheumatologists in the United Kingdom. Although the likelihood of disability is greater with rheumatoid arthritis than osteoarthritis, seven times more people are disabled because of osteoarthritis. At the other end of the spectrum the connective tissue diseases are much rarer and not therefore a public health problem, although they are often associated with considerable mortality, particularly in young people.

Rheumatoid arthritis

Ranking of top three reasons for general practice consultations

	45–64	Age 65–74	≥75
Men	Respiratory	Circulatory	Circulatory
	Musculo-skeletal	Respiratory	Respiratory
	Circulatory	Musculo-skeletal	Musculo-skeletal
Women	Musculo-skeletal	Circulatory	Circulatory
	Respiratory	Musculo-skeletal	Musculo-skeletal
	Mental	Respiratory	Respiratory

Data from third RCGP morbidity survey (OPCS).

This disease affects three times more women than men. It can occur at any age but most commonly in the fourth and fifth decades. Its estimated prevalance is 0.5–1%, which is fairly constant worldwide. Recent reports have suggested that there might be a secular decline and that rates are only half those seen 30 to 50 years previously. Studies of twins have shown only a modest genetic effect, with about 20% concordance in identical female twins, and family studies have shown a threefold increased risk in first degree relatives. Other studies have shown a strong association with the presence of HLA DR4 and DR1, producing a relative risk six times higher.

Environmental factors are therefore likely to be important, although there are few strong associations. Those that have been commonly implicated include a protective effect of the contraceptive pill, parity as opposed to nulliparity, and breast feeding. There is also a curious inverse relationship with schizophrenia. Despite immunological evidence pointing to an infectious trigger, there is little in the way of epidemiological evidence to support this. No clear clustering has been found in incident cases and no links have been found with previous childhood diseases, size of households, or number of siblings.

Mortality is considerable in certain groups. An increased mortality of around two to three times is seen if only those being treated in hospital are considered, although this drops to only a 50% increase when other patients are included. Life table analysis has shown, however, that patients seen in hospital have a worse five year survival rate than age matched cases with Hodgkin's disease or triple vessel cardiovascular disease. In terms of morbidity there is some suggestion that patients are currently less severely affected than they were 30 to 50 years ago. Current estimates are that about a third of patients attending a specialist clinic will be moderately or severely disabled in 10 years, a third will be slightly disabled, and a third will maintain normal function. Patients are at higher risk of developing myelomas and lymphomas, but this does not seem to be related to their underlying treatment.

Osteoarthritis

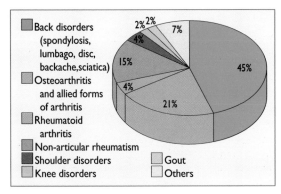

Back disorders (spondylosis, lumbago, disc, backache, sciatica) — 45%
Osteoarthritis and allied forms of arthritis — 21%
Rheumatoid arthritis — 4%
Non-articular rheumatism — 15%
Shoulder disorders — 4%
Knee disorders — 2%
Gout — 2%
Others — 7%

Annual patient consulting rates for arthritic conditions (RCGP morbidity survey)

The prevalance of osteoarthritis (apparent on radiographs) is extremely age dependent. Below the age of 40 less than 5% of people will have any evidence of disease. By the age of 75, however, over 70% will have radiological features of the disease in some parts of their body. Osteoarthritis of the knee is the commonest cause of disability, affecting locomotor function in 10% of the population aged over 50. The disease often first manifests between 45 and 55 in women, in whom disease is two or three times more common than in men.

Osteoarthritis is common worldwide, although the sites most commonly affected vary in different populations. Obesity is the major risk factor for osteoarthritis of the knee, particularly in middle aged women, in whom for every 5 kg increase in weight the risk increases by 30%. Other known risk factors include extensive knee bending and previous knee injuries such as menosectomy. There is also conflicting evidence that weight bearing sports increase the risk.

Osteoarthritis of the hip is less common than that of the knee, but is more likely to cause disability. The prevalence of the disease is only 3% up to age 65, increasing to 10% in people in their 80s. Obesity is not a major risk factor for the hip. However, there are strong occupational associations, such as a fivefold to 10-fold increase in farmers performing long term carrying and lifting. There is also conflicting evidence that acetabular dysplasia is responsible for a percentage of cases.

The heritability of osteoarthritis is currently based on scanty data, although it is likely that hand disease at least is highly genetic— Heberden's nodes of the fingers being found with four to five times the expected frequency in first degree relatives.

The natural course of osteoarthritis is not well understood. By the time patients attend a clinic only about a third will continue to progress radiologically over the next 10 years. Factors affecting progression are unclear but obesity is likely to be the most important factor, at least for the knee, and the presence of Heberden's nodes also seems to identify a high risk group.

Osteoporosis

Approximate number of expected patients with musculoskeletal disease in an average general practice list of 2000 patients aged 18–90

	Women	Men	Total
Chronic back pain	70	70	140
Osteoarthritis	50	30	80
Osteoporosis	50	15	65
Soft tissue rheumatism	10	9	19
Rheumatoid arthritis	10	3	13
Polymyalgia rheumatica	8	2	10
Ankylosing spondylitis	1	6	7
Systemic lupus erythematosus and other connective tissue diseases	1	0	1

The main consequence of osteoporosis is fracture, the most serious being hip fracture, which affects one in four women living to the age of 85, with a lifetime risk of 15%. A quarter of these elderly patients die within a year, and over half remain permanently disabled. The principal risk factors for hip fracture are those that contribute to (a) lack of bone strength, such as early or artificial menopause, family history, smoking, low body weight, being white, female sex, chronic diseases, and use of corticosteroids, and (b) an increase in the risk of falling, including age, postural instability, dementia, lack of muscle strength, and concomitant medication. Genetic factors are believed to be highly important, and studies of twins have shown that these account for up to 70% of the variation in bone density and independent risk. Other predictive factors are history of fracture, family history, and the length of the femoral neck.

Preventive measures include increasing the amount of exercise, reducing cigarette smoking, and maintaining bone density with long term postmenopausal oestrogens and calcium and vitamin D supplements in elderly people.

Back pain

There is a paucity of good epidemiological data on back pain. About 40% of adults will have complained of an episode of back pain in the past year, with 80% reporting ever having had back pain. There is no clear effect of age, and rates are similar in males and females. There are no good data on the genetics of back pain, and environmental risk factors that have been implicated include body height, recent pregnancy, cigarette smoking, depression, low work satisfaction, low social class, and poor education.

Systemic lupus erythematosus

Epidemiology of systemic lupus erythematosus

Prevalence 30/100,000
Incidence 3/100,000
Female to male ratio 9:1
Increase in African-American populations
Commonest age at onset 35–45
High mortality in ethnic minorities
Eightfold risk in first degree relatives

The prevalence of the condition is about 30 cases per 100 000 with increased rates in black people, particularly African Americans, who are at a three to fourfold increased risk. In most populations the disease is nine times commoner in females than males. The commonest age of onset is between 35 and 45 years. All studies have shown an increased mortality, and rates are highest in ethnic minorities and in poor socioeconomic groups. There is a strong genetic contribution—that is, an eightfold increase in risk if you have a first degree relative with the disease and higher rates in identical twins than in non-identical twins. There is a weak association with HLA DR2 and DR3 in white people. Search for other risk factors has been generally unrewarding and there has been no consistent evidence that infection, chemicals, or diet are involved in aetiology. Furthermore, despite the strong effect of sex on the disease, no clear epidemiological evidence exists that reproductive or hormonal factors are important.

Ankylosing spondylitis

Prevalence of ankylosing spondylitis and HLA B27

Ankylosing spondylitis	
White population	1·5/1000
Black Americans	0·4/1000
American Indians	50/1000

HLA B27	
United Kingdom, United States	8–10%
Scandinavia	17%
American Indians	50%

The prevalence in white people is about 1.5 per 1000 and there are clear differences between white and non-white groups. The frequency in black Americans is one quarter that of white people and the disease is rare in Africa and Japan but very high in American Indian indigenous groups. The prevalence of the disease tends to correlate with the prevalence of the genetic marker HLA B27. The frequency of B27 is believed to be 8–10% in the United Kingdom and United States and higher in Scandinavian populations. Over 90% of patients have the B27 marker, although those negative for it often share a common epitope. B27 on its own is obviously not sufficient to cause the disease, and it is likely that an infectious agent acts as a trigger, such as *Klebsiella*, *Shigella*, or *Yersinia*. The disease is believed to be three times commoner in males than females, but if only mild disease is considered the prevalence is equal, with males being prone to more severe disease. It is believed that the mean time from onset of symptoms to radiographic diagnosis is about eight years. The disease has considerable morbidity, although more than 21% are able to continue working normally after 20 years of disease. There is no marked increase in mortality.

Gout

Prevalence of gout

Men	
Average	1–2%
Micronesians	10%
Black Africans	<0·1%
Women	0·2–0·5%

The prevalence of gout varies markedly between different populations. Current estimates in men are between 1–2% and gout is far commoner in men than women in all populations. Rural populations tend to have lower rates than those in towns. The highest rates of gout in the world however, are in Polynesian Islanders; Micronesians from Naura have rates of 10% in men. Black African groups, however, have a complete absence of gout in most studies. There is some evidence that the incidence of gout has increased over the past 30 or 40 years, paralleling an increase in serum uric acid concentrations. The major risk factor for gout is hyperuricaemia with an approximate relationship. Men generally have higher levels of uric acid than women. Other important risk factors include obesity, hypertension, and lead exposure, particularly occupational lead exposure. Alcohol intake has been shown to be associated with uric acid levels, although the relationship with clinical gout is less clear cut in a number of studies. Clear associations have been found with the drinking of "moonshine" whisky and wine stored in lead based containers. Gout itself is not fatal but its association with obesity, hypertension, and coronary artery disease is often indirectly associated with early death.

Polymyalgia rheumatica

Incidence of polymyalgia rheumatica in over 50s

Women   10–50/100 000
Men   5–25/100 000

The exact frequency of this condition is difficult to ascertain, although most estimates put the incidence in the over 50s somewhere between 10 and 50 per 100 000. It is rarely a cause of death. Polymyalgia rheumatica and giant cell arteritis are exceptionally rare in people under the age of 50. The incidence increases dramatically between 6th and 7th decades and declines in the over 80s. It is more common in women at all ages. There is a suggestion that the disease is commoner in the United States and northern Europe and rare in Oriental populations. There is some evidence of clustering within families but large studies are sparse. There is no clear association with genetic markers, or of infectious or environmental influences suggested by apparent clustering of cases in time or space. There is some evidence of seasonal clustering, with most but not all studies showing a summer peak. There is no clear increased death rate due to the disease, although the risk of blindness is increased even in those who have taken corticosteroids.

INDEX

Index

Index

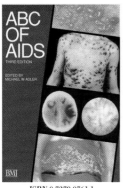
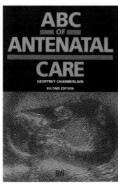
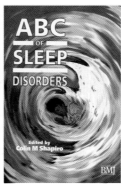
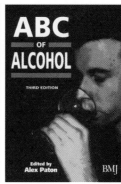
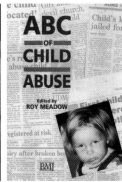
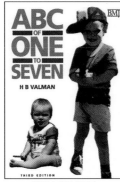
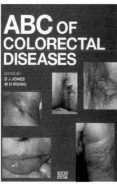
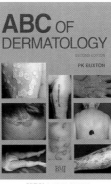
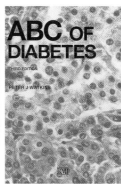
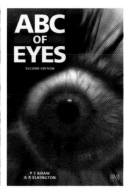
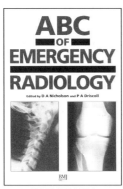
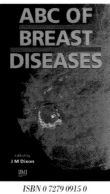
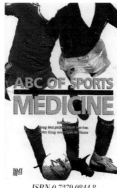
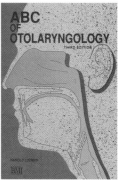
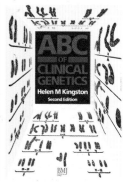
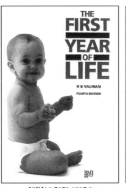
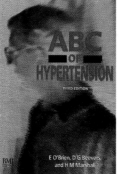
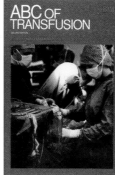
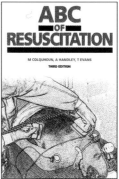
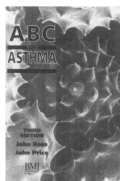
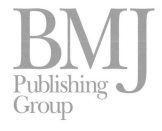